How to be a Good Enough GP

Surviving and thriving in the new primary care organisations

Gerhard Wilke

with

Simon Freeman

Foreword by

Professor Sean Hilton

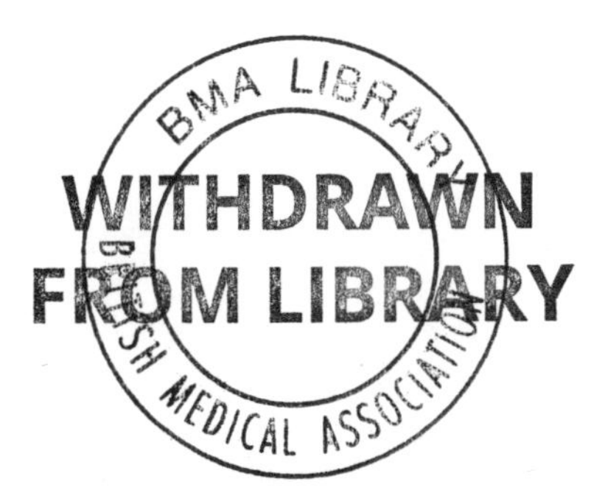

Radcliffe Medical Press

Radcliffe Medical Press Ltd
18 Marcham Road, Abingdon, Oxon OX14 1AA

British Library Cataloguing in Publication Data

A catalogue record for this book is available from the British Library.

ISBN 1 85775 358 5

Typeset by Acorn Bookwork, Salisbury, Wiltshire
Printed and bound by TJ International Ltd, Padstow, Cornwall

Contents

Foreword

Primary care overall, and general practice in particular, face challenging times in coming years. General practitioners within the NHS have endured a decade of reforms and re-organisations throughout the 1990s. These have brought numerous pressures into partnerships and primary healthcare teams, and there is little doubt that the emerging structures of PCGs and PCTs will bring new pressures and tensions.

Whilst many resources will undoubtedly be allocated to change management, organisational development and learning sets, this book offers a different perspective and a challenging approach to understanding and supporting the individuals who make up the primary care workforce.

In the mid-1990s the Department of Health funded a three-year experiment – the London Implementation Zone Educational Initiative scheme (LIZEI) – to address problems of recruitment and retention among the general practice workforce in inner London. The GP workforce overall was reckoned to be stretched, morale was low and recruitment to inner-city practice was difficult. Among other investments in primary care that followed (e.g. the Tomlinson Report on health services in London), the LIZEI scheme funded protected time for GPs to pursue educational activities. One of the more innovative schemes within the programme was the Bolingbroke Project. This enabled GPs in south-west London to join educational groups. In addition to studying clinical issues and educational needs, these small groups held regular sessions led by Gerhard Wilke, a psychoanalyst, to discuss their working environment. They were able to probe and address the pressures that arise from working in such a demanding and unforgiving organisation as the NHS.

In this book, Gerhard Wilke has drawn on his experiences in leading these groups, and also on his extensive experience before and after the LIZEI period, to identify the reason(s) behind the 'dis-ease' felt by many practitioners and to suggest models for improving their morale. As an active participant in the Bolingbroke Project, Simon Freeman gives a GP's perspective, explaining how insights gained from the project have helped him to deal with subsequent NHS changes.

This book will be of interest to practitioners working through the challenges of continuing 'top-down' reorganisation of the NHS and responding to the reconfiguration of general practice partnerships into PCGs and PCTs.

Sean Hilton
Professor of General Practice and Primary Care
St George's Hospital Medical School
University of London
October 2000

About the authors

Gerhard Wilke studied social anthropology at King's College, Cambridge. He spent almost 20 years lecturing in various institutions of higher and further education in London. In the late 1980s he re-trained as a group analyst and psychotherapist and has become a member of the Institute of Group Analysis in London. He has built up organisational consultancy and training programmes based on psychodynamic and group analytic principles in the public and private sector – both in the UK and the rest of Europe. Since the GP Contract in 1990 he has invested a lot of his time and effort into helping GP Partner Groups and primary healthcare teams process the tensions and anxieties involved in accomplishing a series of fundamental changes in their professional world.

The projects Gerhard Wilke has completed during the last decade in primary care include: one-to-one support for single handers and senior partners; a partner and team development programme in a number of health centres; support groups for GPs with complaints pending; a research project designed to explore how much change people will implement when they are not asked to follow imposed reforms from above. In conjunction with St George's Medical School, London he conducted a weekly group designed to help GPs to re-construct their professional identity to cope with the integration of medicine, management and politics in their daily practice lives. This book makes sense of his accumulated experience and passes on the lessons he has learnt about organisational change, strategy, patient care and professional development from this work. It shows GPs how their complex and paradoxical feelings and thoughts during the process of developing or getting stuck in primary care organisations are normal and understandable. The message is both simple and complex: it is legitimate to ask for support and put the needs of the GP alongside those of the patient; doctors need support just as much as other carers and if they want help this book offers ideas on how to get it. One of the key hypothesis put forward here is that self-care is the key to better patient care and healthier primary care organisations.

You can contact Gerhard Wilke at gerhardwilke@compuserve.com

Simon Freeman is a GP working in Battersea, South London. He was actively engaged in the Bolingbroke Project as a facilitator of the groups throughout the three-year period that the LIZEI scheme was operational. He continues to be involved in local initiatives that will support GPs in the context of Battersea Primary Care Group's Clinical Governance Framework.

Chapter	**How to be a Good Enough GP** Surviving and thriving in the new primary care organisations	*Period of change*
1	**The foundation matrix** **Macrosystem** and change GPs – Patients – Society	Past **15** years
2	Microsystem **of the PHCT** Partners – Patients – Staff – NHS	Previous reform but **relevant** to all PHCTs
3	How groups deal with change – Group dynamics	In all work groups
4	How individuals do and do not cope with reforms and imposed change	Everyone at any time
5,6	**Beyond Balint** Change and professional development through supervision and experiential learning	Current reform and in the future
7	A group analytic paradigm of organisations Resolving the conflict between the machine and chaos metaphor	20th and 21st centuries
8	The relevance of the argument to a GP in a PCG moving towards PCT status	Now and in the future

CHAPTER ONE

Dis-ease in primary care: the foundation matrix

The symptoms of trauma and exhaustion

General practitioners display the symptoms of mild trauma and stress under the pressure of coping with a perceived increase in patient demand and a decrease in support from the NHS and government. All primary care reforms since 1990 have generated a groundswell of undigested and unpalatable feelings and thoughts associated with the change process. These regressive forces are bound to be reactivated during the setting up of primary care groups (PCGs) and trusts (PCTs) because individuals and groups who feel pushed around and traumatised try to work through the experience by re-enacting it when a situation arises which unconsciously reminds them of the original trauma. In this book I want to explore where we should locate the problem: in the individual GP, in the system, in our age or in a matrix which connects all these forces of change?

The British psychoanalyst and paediatrician Donald Winnicott wrote that in the early stages of human development we should not envisage a separate baby and mother but only the relationship between them. By this he meant that mental 'wellness' and 'unwellness' are developed in the space between the mother and the child. It is the quality of the relationship built up through their interactions that is internalised by the growing child and used as an inner resource when faced with the task of progressing or regressing in later life. If we apply this idea to the primary care reforms, it is the inner quality of the relationship between the health authority and the GP and the leader of a group and its individual member which will shape how much progress and regression occurs during the process of institutionalising PCGs.

Group analysts locate problems that hinder development in relation to personal development or task performance in the group matrix and foundation matrix of the wider system and not in a pathologised individual. If things don't work, it is the whole group that creates the problem, not a particular, dysfunctional person within it. What groups do is locate the shared problem in one of its members so that this individual can appear to be the problem and the rest of the group can pretend to be healthy. In primary care the projected problem GP is the single-hander. The planners of recent primary care reforms seem to think that if these 'dinosaurs' of general practice could be made to join in a group, the whole system would be more efficient. The unconscious denial involved in this projection is the fear of having to acknowledge that improvements in primary care might not be as measurable, predictable and controllable as current political and management fashions want us to believe. In the primary care system the single-hander is the repository of the secretly desired independence in each frustrated partner in a primary healthcare team (PHCT). Single-handers don't have to put up with partners or overdemanding professional colleagues and are loved by loyal patients who still know about traditional respect and subservience to authority.

By the term 'matrix', group analysts mean the invisible transpersonal network of relationships which hold a group together. The group matrix is characterised by conscious verbal and unconscious non-verbal communication. Gregori van der Kleij (1982) used a helpful image to explain what this might mean when he wrote that the matrix is a sentence, each group member is a word and the group process gives meaning to the structure of the sentence. Group analysts see the 'dis-ease' displayed by an individual unable or unwilling to engage with changes as a symptom of unease in the whole group. All groups have this built-in mechanism. By resisting the temptation to blame the individual and by relocating the problem in the shared matrix, symptoms of resistance can be treated as a communication. The symptom is telling the group and its leader a story about the task that needs to be taken on and worked through. Each group has a matrix unique to the individuals connected within this network. Together they will live through the normal stages of group forming, storming, norming and ending but each matrix will have to do it in its own way. The different group matrices are, in turn, invisibly connected to a foundation matrix that contains elements of cultural, historical and social memory which make up the system or the organisation. I would call this the social unconscious.

A shared humanity unites and distinct professional identities divide

Primary care is formed by the interactions between the unconscious mind of each PCG and the social unconscious of the NHS foundation matrix. This foundation matrix symbolises the shared culture, the history and the current political and economic preoccupations of the NHS and the society in which it is embedded. To use an image from gestalt thinking: the foundation matrix forms the base of our shared common humanity and the group matrix lends us a distinct cultural and professional identity. The NHS is so big that the study of society in general is relevant to an understanding of how the system works for the people within it. Modern social anthropologists like Edmund Leach (1986) have come to the conclusion that we share a species identity common to us all but that we are also group animals and need differentiation, 'structuration' and boundaries. We seem to feel normal only if each tribe or each professional group knows 'who we are' and also 'who they are'. We tend to determine our own self-worth by denigrating our neighbours, the other uniprofessional group, as worthless or inferior to us. If I am in a PCG containing only ex-fundholders, I might think that I am one step closer to being a PCT and don't have to waste my time and energy on improving a group full of single-handers and non-fundholders, who I am used to perceiving as resisters and premodernists. The rivalry between doctors and nurses is simply another version of the pattern of denigration and idealisation that all cultural groups use to negotiate their relationship to each other and define the boundaries between them.

Mutual idealisation and denigration have set the tone in the relationship between reforming managers and reluctant GPs over the last decade. These splits into goodies and baddies, insiders and outsiders are also set in concrete between the unidisciplinary subgroups in most PHCTs. However, the segregation between professionals remains unnamed in the overly optimistic universe of the multidisciplinary team. I would argue that the very existence of culture depends on 'us' re-creating the meaning of 'our belonging' and 'our enemy group' through daily interaction between 'us' and with 'them'. Culture with a capital C exists neither in society nor in primary care. The primary care culture is more rooted in the social unconscious than in the norms, values and visions of the organisation which get written down in the strategy and fixed in an organisational chart. In other words, the PCG comes into existence when it actually meets and engages in social intercourse: before that it is an abstract idea.

From this way of looking at an organisation it follows that the success of a reform such as the introduction of PCGs depends literally on the quality and patterns of interaction that take place when its members meet. It is during the face-to-face meeting that the members of the PCG accomplish their business but also re-create the 'illusion' of the group's existence. If a culture of direct and open communication can be developed within clearly defined boundaries and a visible structure of hierarchy and role differentiation, then a cultural matrix can be woven which will be strong enough to deal with the stresses and strains of change. This culture of relatedness in everyday life is more important than management toolkits and procedure documents. Whether this culture can be created depends, ultimately, on the sum of the unconscious early childhood experiences of the group's members.

Unlearning and relearning the GP role

Let me now ask what kind of psychic forces and cultural factors are forming the ground (the foundation matrix) on which the latest primary care reform takes shape. The current GP acts as a location point in the primary care foundation matrix between vocation and modernisation. During this journey of transition, losing a secure sense of professional identity and having to construct another, each GP is confronted with the unlearning and relearning of the meaning attached to the medical role.

> One might say that the learning of the medical role consists of a separation, almost an alienation, of the student from the lay medical world; a passing through the mirror so that one looks out on the world from behind it, and sees things in mirror writing. (Everett Hughes, 1984)

Medical training has made it difficult for GPs to be at ease in groups and a key to making PCGs work will be the willingness of the government and PCG managers to invest in the development of group skills among GPs and other health professionals. Doctors are socialised into an overdeveloped sense of self-reliance and responsibility, which makes team membership and the sharing of power and professional interdependence difficult. The professional training of doctors has also left them with a legacy of idealising patient care and denigrating management and politics. Most damaging of all is the tradition of always putting the patient first and never having any prior claim to care and attention. Survival and recreation in the current context of continuous change and improvement depend on whether the doctor can learn that self-care is the best way to improve patient care.

Globalisation in the world economy could be described as the politicisation of manufacture and trade and the NHS reforms of the last 15 years have, attendant upon this larger transformation, led to the politicisation of primary care. Before PCGs can succeed, old professional ideals and ways of seeing the world have to be given up, separated from and mourned. Many years after training and before each primary care reform, the GP is in a hall of mirrors reflecting back distorted images of other people's expectations. In the primary care hall of distorting mirrors the unconscious projections of the key players are collected and anyone who looks straight will notice that those who care about general practice have different and partially overlapping and conflicting expectations of each other and the service. The result is severe role strain and chronic exhaustion.

The mirror is a favoured psychoanalytic metaphor designed to capture some of the unconscious and collusive relationships between therapist and patient in a one-to-one relationship and between different members of a group. The mirror metaphor was used by Balint to capture the unconscious interaction between doctor and patient; it is a way of reflecting on the dynamic interaction between the self and the other in a significant relationship. In common-sense terms, mirroring could be viewed as giving and receiving feedback. Here I want to apply the metaphor of mirroring to GPs, the health authority, the members of PCGs and the patients, who all re-create the system through their daily interactions and the exchange of their wishes and needs. The mirror is a mutual 'projection' screen that serves to identify the outlines of the psychic interdependence of doctor and manager, doctor and patient, doctor and staff, PCG and political system. The 'projective identification' is interactive and together the social actors in the primary care world form a psychological matrix (invisible and at least half unconscious network of relationships) in which they are the location points for each other's ideals, problems, and split-off and unwanted parts.

Together primary care teams, secondary care providers and the whole NHS are one projection screen for the rest of society, which expects medical carers and doctors to collude with its wish to deny death and illness. Patients and politicians in our society now expect the doctor/magician to overcome the unfair ways in which death and misfortune interfere with an ideal lifeplan by waving a magic wand and never making any mistakes. If this fails, a customer care-led complaints system ensures that the offending magician is publicly shamed and the offence is neutralised by a revision of procedures. The new PCGs offer doctors a chance to take back some of the power and leadership which they need if they are to discharge their responsibilities to the patients in a mature and non-magical way.

Helpless rage and the destruction of ideals

The often socially dislocated patient with very high expectations in today's primary care world, like the stepmother in Snow White, consults the mirror on the wall (the doctor's face) to look for reassurance and relief from inner anxiety. Many patients hope at the beginning of the consultation that nothing has changed, that they are still predominantly in a narcissistic relationship with an ideal self, with a healthy body and the eternal youth required by the media ideal of the beautiful people to whom they want to belong. When the mirror tells the patient that the fantasy world has changed and that the body is now less than perfect, they feel deeply outraged. Like a little child who has discovered that the parents are less than perfect, the 'problem' patient defends against an inner loss of security and the resultant fears of disintegration by raging against fate. They try to reintegrate a fragmenting sense of self through aggression against an envied object possessing the privileges they have apparently lost: that object is the GP. The doctor is made to feel how little a GP can really do against the inevitable decline of the body and loses a sense of a perfect medical order. Even worse, the problem patient might be mirroring how the GP feels inside about the never-ending series of primary care reforms which have destroyed his or her own self-ideal as a doctor who is never challenged, is always in control and is never offended. The heart-sink patient is outraged in the face of losing his imagined perfect body, the doctor is helpless and full of inner rage in the face of losing an ideal way of doing general practice.

Before each primary care reform doctors and other health professionals have processed the loss of a treasured way of working like a problem patient and displayed similar symptoms. This was particularly true of the new GP Contract in 1990. When this reform had to be accepted, many GPs regressed to a childlike state and, like the problem patient, fought against the unfair destruction of their cherished professional health. Snow White's change from a dependent child into a mature sexual rival drove her stepmother into murderous rage and a lust for revenge and persecution. The loss of the perfect doctor role, ideally in sole command of the primary care world, left many GPs with similarly primitive emotions. To relieve themselves of their inner rage, they acted like their worst patients and wanted revenge, looked for self-destruction or sought to escape by giving up on the profession.

Politicians and the mid-life crisis of the good GP

The Thatcherite reforms smashed the traditional relationship between doctor and government which was based on a fantasy of eternal harmony and maternal provision. The change shattered the GP's vocational ideal of just wanting to be a good carer by being a good doctor: a good doctor being a GP who concentrates on real cases, real medicine and real patients. Malingerers, false presenters and community care cases ought to have a hospital bed or be cared for by someone else. The changes demanded of GPs were experienced as a terrible 'narcissistic injury' and many of them were lost for a way out of the vale of tears in primary care. They descended individually, and as a profession, into a profound mid-life crisis: the pain of the transition is still at the core of the experience of being a doctor in a PCG. Those most eager to embrace the reform might not really be converts to the politics of primary care but are simply acting out a defence against further loss of security by being a compliant child or by taking back control. The majority of the older GPs would much rather return to the good old days of doctoring, without audit, reaccreditation, quality control and best value.

Illness is for patients, permanent health and improvement are for GPs

The reforms of the last decade made a return to the golden age of primary care impossible and left many GPs feeling attacked, abandoned and rejected. They felt subjected to a barrage of persecutors, with the government in alliance with consumers and the media. The doctors felt that the NHS had turned from a supportive and nurturing 'environmental mother' into a failing and persecuting parent who had begun to put her own needs before those of the dependent children (Winnicott, 1965). The NHS as the parent forced the GP into an enforced growing-up process by demanding financial self-management, health promotion targets and managerial 'empowerment'. The system drew a rigid boundary between its responsibilities to the government and patients and its willingness and ability to be a prop for the GP and PHCT. When support came, it was offered when the reform itself was way off target and needed to be rescued.

Support and development began to be perceived as a cynical exercise, not a genuine opportunity. The GP became a grown-up subcontractor solely responsible for preserving a professional integrity, keeping up the morale of the practice team and delivering a good service to patients. The primary care reforms have assumed that the personal resources of the GP, available to the patients, are limitless and can be made more bountiful year by year. The doctor who looks after the sick, so the taken-for-granted logic of a continuous improvement programme implies, never needs care or support. Illness is for patients, permanent health is for doctors. A problem-free and electronically administered practice is what the system expects the doctor to present in an audit to the policy-makers.

A few years ago many GPs felt like giving up their cherished careers or developed symptoms of stress and burn-out. Instead of working their way out of the helpless victim position by developing a more proactive attitude towards management, patients and politics, doctors regressed in the face of progress. In fact, doctors exposed their own need for support and care through their response to the political demands made on them in recent years.

Helper syndrome

The internal, psychological inability to respond to change in a rational way in primary care is tied up with the overidealised doctor–patient relationship which hides the fact that many GPs suffer from what psychoanalysts have called helper syndrome (Schmidbauer, 1993). Helping is often a form of altruistic self-sacrifice designed to hide an inner emptiness and lack of confidence in the carer. The helping doctor has often ended up in the profession by fulfilling parental wishes and spent a lifetime complying with other people's expectations in order to obtain the necessary qualifications and skills. The length and depth of this resocialisation programme have produced a type of doctor who is not consciously in touch with their true self and can only present a false self to the patient, manager or staff. Deep down this person feels that there is a 'basic fault' in their own personality, but admission of this fact evokes a fear of being overwhelmed by one's own needs (Balint, 1973). It is infinitely preferable to go on unconsciously recapturing a part of the true self in the doctor–patient relationship by finding the needy child and the damaged self in the patient who is defined as treatable and deserving of attention. After years of practice at this indirect way of getting in touch with their innermost needs, desires and aggression via the patient, the GP has lost the capacity for being in a relationship based on mutual exchange and interdependence.

When a person with a helper mindset is confronted by change which demands an engagement on an adult-to-adult level, the demand will initially expose the inability to do so spontaneously. If the demand is enforced it will strengthen the false self and drive the true self, which is the only resource for change anyone has, completely underground. The diagnostic picture of helper syndrome is then thrown into stark relief: an inability to trust in others, resentful performance of duties, withdrawn behaviour, increased difficulty in defining what the self needs and a fear of open and direct communication and conflict. Any talk of partnership and healthy alliances, which the health authorities developed after the 1990 Contract, remained just talk and increased the level of cynicism and resentment. Similar feelings were expressed in a support group which I ran when primary care pilots were set up. Even in this group of enthusiasts, the common ground was that they had to go along with the change introduced by New Labour. With very few exceptions, the group would have preferred a period of stability and consolidation. If they had been given a choice they would, without doubt, have voted for a postponement of this radical reform.

From fear of annihilation to survival and re-creation

Larry Hirschhorn (1993) argued that people have a workplace without and within. In the workplace within we process the psychodynamic forces which underlie organisational life and get anxious about the relationships to our bosses, the task and the organisation as a belonging group. The organisations we work for can make us safe by becoming a carer substitute or threaten our integrity by making demands that we feel exceed our inner resources. Hirschhorn shows that we are task oriented and anxious at the same time. Work groups manage their anxiety about the measurement of their performance by developing social defences. Social defences distort outcomes and professional relationships and represent a retreat from the task, clear boundaries and role differentiation. These social defences can also undermine the relationship of a professional group to the organisational reality beyond itself. The outside is devalued and scapegoated to preserve a fragile and fragmented 'I' and 'we' identity within the group.

Professional groups in a social defence position retreat from the boundary with the rest of the organisation into a fantasy world of control and safety from change. The desire to defend against anxiety is connected with a desire to repair the damage caused by imposed change; it is an attempt to restore wholeness of the person, the 'we' identity of our belonging group and the confidence of the professional self which feels shattered inside.

The process of undermining the integrity of the GP's professional self started with the creation of multidisciplinary teams. Although this change made sense and is generally accepted in primary care, it nevertheless caused feelings of loss and disorientation which were never faced by doctors who were the main losers in this restructuring of their organisational world. What was an orderly world of primary care reflecting traditional, patriarchal structures with clearly defined roles, a division of labour and a hierarchical view of power and responsibility was reversed and levelled. Shared rather than divided tasks made team members more equal and responsible on paper. Internally this blurring of boundaries caused increased anxiety that found release in a culture of blame rather than mutual understanding. The structures were more transparent but the degree of anxiety about status and security made people so tense that they ended up with even less understanding of the experience of those in roles other than their own.

A good example of this was the creation of nurse practitioners. On paper an excellent idea, in reality this measure increased the workload of doctors in the short term. As the boundaries between the GP and the nurse became blurred it was no longer clear who had to do the boring bits of nursing. Instead of distributing the workload more rationally, I saw this well-intentioned reform increase the intergroup tension between GPs, traditional nurses and nurse practitioners. Instead of sorting out the joint ownership of the workload, nurse practitioners projected their increased demands on the system onto the doctors and blamed them for an apparent lack of support. Equally, the doctors projected their own difficulties finding a new role as a GP, staff coach and politician onto the nurse practitioners by expecting them to take up the new role without proper socialisation into it. The reform did not make the PHCT more equal and flat but produced symbolic patterns of sibling rivalry, fratricide and matricide. I have no reason to believe that the multifunctional management boards in PCGs will solve this problem without a lot of process work. People who have lost something will regress temporarily to a more primitive psychological way of being and relating. In such a state of mind, dialogue is replaced by scapegoating and blame.

The nurse practitioner scheme was symptomatic of the current organisational context in primary care. We are in a period of transition from a known to an unknown world of work organisation in primary care and those involved feel exposed to the risk of losing familiar roles and the organisation as a psychological home. It is difficult to experience a sense of wholeness in primary care; it is easier to retain a sense of security within an apparently chaotic organisation by dividing the world into perpetrators, victims and bystanders. Working in primary care is currently connected with the feeling of being threatened with disintegration. The underlying fear of each professional group is annihilation, the underlying hope is survival, the task is re-creation on an individual and collective level.

Social defences against anxiety caused by uncertainty

When children grow up they face up to a disappearing world every night at bedtime because they cannot be sure whether the world will still be there when they wake up, nor can they be certain whether they will survive the ordeal of going to sleep without Mummy being there. In this process of developing into a separate human being capable of coping with the challenges of growing up, the child resorts to using a teddy bear. Winnicott called this toy a transitional object that helps the child master the anxiety involved in being independent and trusting in the world. The transitional object exists half outside the child and half in his or her mind. Psychoanalysts looking at organisations have also seen work as a transitional object. Work can thus be a reparative force, which helps the adult to be a social being dependent on self-respect, a connection to the social world and in need of feedback and recognition. Work is a means of having these needs fulfilled and accepted in a structured, orderly and confirming way.

Hirschhorn (1993) has taken this image and argued that we need to conceptualise work as a transitional object to help us accomplish the transition from a culture of social defences to a culture of development and learning. Only a learning and developmental culture can, in his view, help us cope with the sense of unknowing which is now a constituent part of organisational life. Unlike management consultants and managers, he doesn't reduce this to the introduction of postgraduate training schemes, appraisal and upskilling programmes. Instead, Hirschhorn advises that the development of the human resource should be done through experiential learning which focuses on the needs of the whole human being. He predicts that the incantation of the need to grow up will not produce what the organisational reformers want. People who have been empowered in a human resource development programme will not necessarily end up feeling more responsible simply by being restructured, re-formed, retrained and reconceptualised. They might feel more infantilised and react like recalcitrant children who have displayed their compliant self to the organisation but not internalised any new models of being, working and surviving. When this happens the objects of change in any organisation, including primary care, will retreat from co-operation and resort to a splitting culture to defend against the anxiety caused by an overdemanding organisational parent.

In this context the unconscious collusive systems described by Hirschhorn will take over and undermine the planned changes in an organisation. He identified three social defences against too much anxiety in an organisation: first, basic group defences against an overdemanding task list which he called dependency, splitting and subgrouping; second, covert coalition and collusion; third, rituals designed to prevent effectiveness. An example of dependency is when a group in primary care becomes entirely leader oriented and loses the capacity for independent thought and action. We all know examples from history when this has happened and the group is subservient to a charismatic leader who becomes increasingly manic as the followers project their need for magical solutions on to the messiah who is waiting to become the sacrificial lamb. Splitting is a basic defence against a fear of annihilation (Hopper, 1999). In primary care this is demonstrated when a practice closes ranks against the outside world and declares all patients and health managers to be enemies. When this loss of reality occurs, it is imperative for the group to abandon its sense of individuality and support a leader figure who is ready to fight for the cause of splitting the group into good insiders, bad outsiders and potential traitors. This type of leader is doomed but only after a self-destructive phase in the group.

Subgrouping can be a defence against too much change too fast but it can also be a symptom of group size. The most effective size for a well-functioning work group is eight; anything above that number produces large group phenomena where the rational capacity of each of its members is significantly impaired by underlying anxieties about the group devouring its children. In this situation group members defend themselves by overidentifying with a distinct subgroup; people look for safety in numbers. Many PHCTs and all PCGs will be larger than a benign work group of eight and I would predict that the social defences identified by Hirschhorn will determine its work unless clear leadership structures are created. In one health authority, anxiety about the introduction of PCGs reached such levels that the GP population in the area split into ethnic subgroups. The GPs in their religiously based affiliation groups transferred their basic mistrust of the health authority onto their colleagues and formed defence leagues, lest the health authority conspire to appoint yet another set of change leaders who would sell them down the river.

Social anthropologists noticed that during periods of transition groups tend to fall victim to moral panics which can only be calmed by a restatement of the cosmological order and a ritualised re-enactment of the boundaries between subgroups. Only when the panicking group is reconnected with a sense of belonging does it recover a basic sense of trust in its own ability to stay sane and engage in a constructive way with the problems of everyday life. A classic case of this in a group that one can assume shares the same interests is an extended family when somebody has died. The period of mourning is regulated by many ritualistic prescriptions and the large group of those bereft is divided into family and relatives. Family equates with insiders, relatives with outsiders. Family are blood related and can, in periods of uncertainty, be trusted blindly. Relatives are acquired by marriage and represent, in uncertain times, the enemy within.

Waves of primary care reform compare to periods of mourning and moral uncertainty. It made sense that the GPs should split themselves into subgroups of potential friends and enemies before engaging in the process of forming and institutionalising PCGs. They acted in accordance with cultural patterns which are as old as humanity itself and by so doing, they let the primary care system know that reform intentions are one thing, reform outcomes quite another.

The best example of covert coalitions as a defence against change that I have come across has been the unconscious 'pairing' of a castrated senior partner and the practice manager against the young modernisers. The young champions of change had succeeded in preventing the normal succession based on age and seniority but had failed to elect a *primus inter pares*. Consequently, their sibling rivalry displaced power and responsibility onto the practice manager who was the severest judge of performance in the group but the least able to help the PHCT make the transition from the old to the new world of primary care. In reality, neither the young reformers nor the senior partner (shortly before his retirement) wanted to carry the responsibility of transforming a comfortable and known way of working into an uncertain and unpredictable way of organising their team in line with the wishes of the health authority. The whole team got stuck and it needed an outside consultant to move it on by handing the father role back to the older partner and letting him use his wisdom to share authority through a new division of management which reflected the talents and interests of each partner.

The most widespread displacement of conflict within primary care is the perennial problem of absent or lost files. The partners, the practice manger, the administration and the receptionists are all involved in a collusive and ritualised enactment of the hatred and fear of paperwork. No one wants the responsibility for making the system work. Everyone is unconsciously interested in having the system fail, as this proves that the paper mountain which comes with the new primary care world is not worth having and that it would be much better to go back to the old world where records just didn't matter so much. Within the newly created PCGs it is possible that a lot of time will be invested in the creation of a paper reality, an administrative illusion of achievement, in order to hide the conflicts which smoulder underneath the surface, stopping the group from really working.

Reparation and growth in a runaway world

Unconscious forces in a group working against task performance and change implementation are considerable. Let us now look at what a positive list might look like, a list of psychodynamic forces which help change processes and improve performance. Just as we can rely on human psychology to undermine task performance, so we can rely on the same 'drives' to seek reparation and improvement in a situation. To achieve any self-worth, we depend on positive feedback from others and therefore want to do things that are helpful or please others. In return, we get confirmation of the fact that we are decent and good human beings and experience relief from social anxiety by being accepted as valuable members of a work group. Primary care rests on this symbolic gift exchange between help givers and help seekers.

Sigmund Freud has taught us that guilt is a civilising force that acts as a defence against barbarity and disorder in everyday life. Guilt feelings are generated every time it becomes obvious that a primary care member or group has attacked the system and refused the request of an authority figure to comply with the demand to be good. These, in turn, produce a need for reparation to invoke forgiveness and acceptance. Hirschhorn argues that here lies the potential salvation for the individual, the group and the whole organisation in the current context, which Anthony Giddens (1999) in his Reith lectures, 'A Runaway World', has described as a pervasive culture of endings in which there are no beginnings. What Giddens implies by this is that the past is no longer a guide to the future in politics, society and organisations. It is logical that each PHCT and PCG has to continuously reinvent itself whilst simultaneously doing its real job. It mirrors what is happening globally. We have lost the ideas of what Giddens calls the first phase of modernisation, which provided us with a linear, organised and constructed sense of the future. Organisations used to run like clockwork, reflecting the workings of a machine, and careers were made up of predictable steps and lasted for a lifetime. In the globalised order, of which the new primary care structure is one piece in a worldwide jigsaw, unpredictability, manufactured uncertainty, risk taking and fragmentation are the key words. Organisations are no longer seen as machines but are conceptualised as 'bounded chaos', complexity and a continuous process of survival and re-creation.

We first learn about survival and re-creation in the relationship between baby and mother. Hirschhorn points out that the modern world of enforced maturity in organisations mirrors experiences from very early childhood and people affected by such changes react on the basis of their earliest experiences of mothering. If the 'change child' is made safe and its anxieties recognised and contained by a good enough organisational parent, it will retain a sense of self-worth and be able to respond to increased demands in an adult position. Before that, resistance and regression are normal during a period of transition. In this phase the person asked to grow up and change will attack the demanding parent and reject well-meaning advice. However, a person with sufficient ego strength will retain an interest in being related and connected. Such a person wants to remain a member of a belonging group and starts to feel sorry for the act of aggression. At that point the aggressive energy will turn into a need for reparative work which usually takes the form of resolving conflict, solving problems and volunteering for co-operative projects.

When the 'change child' has had a bad experience of mothering, is made insecure and feels 'unheld' during the change process, it regresses and will attack the demand made upon it. Resistance to change in a group dominated by such an individual will take on the form of borderline phenomena. The group will feel quite disturbed and require the intervention of an outside consultant to work through the paralysis. It is very important that GPs take responsibility for the process work that is required to make their PCGs work. My experience has taught me that doctors prefer to be given the resources for process work by the health authority and avoid the need for planning for it in their own budgets. Unconsciously, this amounts to a child setting up the parents to prove that they still love the child. If the support is withheld it demonstrates that the child is justified in feeling abandoned.

Two conflicting organisational paradigms

It is my experience that the health authority managers cling to the machine metaphor of organisations where they look to control, predictability and rational planning when they have created structures which are based on a process model. The GPs experience this as a 'double-bind' message. They should be process oriented and they should have everything under control. Just as language loses its clear meaning when we use mixed metaphors, so organisational processes become confusing when conflicting paradigms are used to structure and manage organisations. I see GPs caught up in a battle between two conflicting organisational paradigms. GPs will, at present, look in vain for adequate support from the primary care reformers, as they seem to think that grown-up professionals should be able to cope with what is demanded of them without additional support to process the feelings generated by the change. It will be a good investment if GPs in PCGs plan to spend enough resources on process work in order to learn from their experience of change and reassert their leadership of primary care.

Organisations, like cultures and families, need a type of creation myth to hold the people in them together. The traditional view is that there were founding parents and that ever since then things have been stable, predictable and safe. Moreover, the inhabitants of an organisation assumed that their mental picture of it should hold for a lifetime. Now chaos and complexity constitute the prevalent metaphors for describing organisational life. The mythic stories of chaotic patterns, structural instability in opposition to functional structures and stable boundaries are the supposed mental holding frames in present-day organisations. In primary care, the problem clients visiting GPs in increasing numbers since the introduction of community care disturb our ideal view of the organisational world – our 'should-be' perspective. Heart-sink patients embody the repressed disturbance in all of us when we, like them, feel that our inner world is no longer holding together. These patients mirror in their symptoms the 'is' world of everyday life in the primary care organisations as it is experienced and perceived. The heart-sink patients in primary care enact or present in their 'dis-ease' the repressed reality of feelings which cannot be named, touched and accepted and must be made unconscious. The function of this form of institutional repression of truth is to preserve the dominant forms of political and managerial dialogue and maintain the fantasy of progress and modernisation within primary care.

In my view organisations like the NHS go on reproducing the split between an imagined whole and fragmenting organisational world. There is still, after a decade of profound change, a subconscious assumption that the centre of the primary care world should hold as in normal times and that things only tend to fall apart when the 'times are out of joint'. In other words: change is pathological, stability is healthy. The new public managers in primary care sing from the same hymn sheet: we need to abandon an idealised, stable organisation and separate from the wish to have only well-behaved patients in the waiting room and supporting managers in the health authority. GPs must accept the volatility of the organisational and social environment and the true range of disturbance in the patient population and dislocation in the primary care system. So must the reformers and managers. It is crucial to get away from either/or scenarios where patients are typecast as curable or untreatable, as naughty or nice; where managers are for or against us; where GPs are old-fashioned or modern. We need to stop thinking in terms of the organisational setting as holding or fragmenting, as populated by cowboys and Indians, and thinking of ourselves as victims or perpetrators. Instead, we must start to see the organisation as something which can be a holding environmental mother and a force of death and fragmentation at the same time and in the same space.

In my experience organisational consultants and managers still cling to the basic assumption that the organisation and the people in it should be predictable, controllable and rational enough to cope with the task and any change process that comes along. In primary care this unquestioned attitude produces managers who have split off their own anxiety about change and projected it into the fantasy that our organisation should embark on a shining path of permanent modernisation. Anyone not falling within that vision is a counter-revolutionary and needs to be overcome, re-educated or medicalised. The insistence on rationality and predictability in organisations is a defence against the threat posed by the unknown and the death-like force of chaos. It is necessary to separate from the model that the world is either functional or dysfunctional and adopt a view that encompasses the integration of the forces of order and disorder, reconnection and fragmentation. The patient, doctor, manager, other carers and the system as a whole can learn to use a crisis to generate a new perspective of the shared task. We must remind ourselves of how easy it is to deny reality and give in to wishful thinking. To hold PCGs together we must start by not wishing the crisis, the hole in the budget or the unreliable system and patients away and learn to deal with the work in a pragmatic and de-idealised way.

Integration and fragmentation in the primary care world

There is a postmodernist perspective on the conflict between chaos and order in organisations. In psychoanalysis the postmodernist view is rooted in the work of Lacan (Bowie, 1991). From a postmodernist perspective the idea that the centre of a person, the matrix of an organisation or a PCG should hold and prevent fragmentation is a false, modernist delusion. Postmodernist thinkers celebrate the dissolution of the core self and a holding cultural centre. Such theorists believe that any idea of an integrated or coherent self or core culture and organisation is an ideological construction, which serves as a defence against the terrifying nature of modernity and its implied instability and fragmentation. Modernity means a crisis of identity; the disembowelment of secure identities is normal. The way out of this crisis is not a return to a Utopian vision of a true and integrated professional self and a holding and motherly organisational environment but the acceptance of fragmentation as the core experience of modernity. We must learn, according to these thinkers, that there is no depth to experience, all is presentation of aspects of self in a variety of social contexts. In this view, the people we label as schizoid are the truest expression of existential reality.

The widespread loss of a coherent professional self among GPs, a holding NHS environment and containing boundaries in primary care do not simply signify modernity but have resulted from the ideological hegemony of globalisation and new public management methods. The losses resulting from these changes must be mourned as they represent a separation from a quality of safety that is no longer there but, at the same time, these changes offer an opportunity for engaging in processes of recovery and reparation. I would argue that we have to engage with the central problem in modernity: we develop a core self in our period of infancy but then have to face the re-creation of this individual self by engaging periodically with a changed reality and readjusting the fit between inside and outside. By forging new relationships and finding other ways of co-operating across jealously guarded professional boundaries, we can survive the organisational upheavals. By making connections we begin to extend and transform our own sense of self-worth and the nature of our professional practice. The difficult patients and the re-engineering managers present such a challenge in our organisations. I feel that we can discover more fitting strategies for coping with disturbed clients, struggling PCGs and visioning managers only by linking up with the matrix of the whole NHS institution. By accepting our dependency within an organisation we re-create a holding environment in the mind and avoid an incestuous retreat from the unknown into our private and overidealised consulting room.

Reform enthusiasts and disturbed patients are two sides of the same coin

Eating disorders are diseases symbolic of our age. Not accidentally, perhaps, the language of the change managers in our organisations mirrors the symptoms. We talk of a lean organisation, we impose or suffer cuts, we are overfed with and sick of change messages and deep down many professionals prefer career suicide and retention of cherished ideals to organisational survival. Many GPs who feel overwhelmed by the massive and imposed change in primary care over the last 10 years have resembled the paralysed and fretting anorexic or the panicking bulimic, doggedly contemplating staying stuck. There is some mileage in looking at people who are unable to deal with change creatively as being unconsciously fused with the organisation as a mother figure. This organisation-as-mother has stopped being nurturing and attuned to the needs of her children and turned into a malignant monster which is filling them up with projections of her own needs. Unable to separate from a loved object and an idealised past and too angry to feel sad, such members of an organisation regress into the position of the helpless baby who compensates for the loss by developing a compliant and false self. The matrix of restructured and re-engineered organisations often displays a paranoid-schizoid quality at the core of its new culture. Staff relate to the organisation in the victim position as a defence against the waves of imposed change and unconsciously experience the institutional holding environment as unsafe and persecutory. Staff begin to act like the self-depriving adolescent who is defending against an unsafe environmental mother by regressing into an eating disorder to retain a sense of control and fend off the total annihilation of their obscured self.

The relationship between most organisations and their staff is in a state of 'dis-ease' and the dialogue between senior managers and staff has been punctured by autistic taboo zones which cannot be brought into a dialogue but get pushed into the deeper recesses of the collective unconscious. I would suggest that the disturbed patients, the disturbing manager and the 'deaf' GP in primary care not only bring their fragmented sense of self into the primary care world but they also enact a sense of disturbance in the organisation and in society. They can dramatise for us how paranoid, manic and persecuted we sometimes feel inside a changing organisation and thereby create a potential space in which a shared rather than fragmented matrix can be re-created within a foundation matrix which is experienced as chaotic and unsafe. The precondition for this is the acceptance of joint responsibility for the losses, the need for change and the desire for safety.

Modern visions: non-hierarchical teams, equal groups, eternal youth and health

When group analysts talk of the matrix they mean the family and the group analytic therapy group. I have applied the term metaphorically to capture the invisible network of relationships and mutual projections that hold people together or split them apart in the primary care world. Foulkes (1986), the founder of group analysis, linked his idea of the group matrix to that of a foundation matrix in an attempt to capture the idea that each matrix is invisibly connected with a metamatrix which is historical, cultural and social. He developed this idea out of Norbert Elias' work on the civilising process. Elias (1978) was particularly interested in how a society becomes civilised or decivilised over long historical periods and showed how, since the Renaissance, these processes have resulted in changed forms of egointegration and superego function. Clifford Geertz (1993), one of the current gurus in social anthropology, thinks about culture in this way and says that we all live suspended in a web of meaning that we create through social interaction. A collection of such webs of meaning constitutes culture which is a phenomenon that is not fixed in time and space but is continually remade and preserved by people re-enacting its meaning in their various group contexts.

If this line of reasoning captures some of the complexity of how social order is re-created, then it makes sense to look at some of the psychological phenomena which stand out in the foundation matrix of our times and see how they unconsciously influence the world of primary care. Christopher Lasch (1979) argued that we now live in the age of narcissism. In organisations this has led to the denigration of parental models of management, the search for flat teams and the delusion of eternal youth and ever-increasing efficiency. The narcissistic condition in the culture also leads to the denial of dependency needs in managers and rage in change leaders against organisational behaviour that refuses to comply with the ideal vision of how work ought to be done. We see glimpses of the rage of the collective narcissist when things go wrong in community care and there is a moral panic demanding that no psychotic in the community will ever kill anybody again. It is these forms of modern delusions that we need to confront. In their own need to institutionalise the profession, doctors have colluded with omnipotent fantasies and promised outcomes which cannot be achieved with certain patient groups. They must return to a sense of realism and start to disillusion the managers and reformers who insist on setting ideal and unreachable targets by pointing out that death, illness, accidents and vulnerability are part of normal life. Bion (1961) argued that thinking, holding, integration and dialogue depend on the ability to tolerate frustration and hatred to a point where we can resist the temptation to act out what we fear. It is wise to allow our disturbed patients to put us in touch with the depth of our fear of madness as individuals, professionals and organisations.

A second cultural strand in the foundation matrix in which organisations are embedded is the resurgence of charismatic leaders in organisations and in society. We now hold training workshops to identify visionary leaders who can deconstruct a whole organisation and its history, find a new mission statement and lead everyone together into the Promised Land. It is ironic that at the end of the century which saw the emergence of the dictator and the crowd as the most potent and destructive political force, we forget the lessons and return to such models of leadership and 'followership'. What all this means is that there is a deep unease in the face of overwhelming and life-threatening forces like globalisation and new public management. In such states of disconnectedness the central thesis of Freud's book on mass psychology and ego development still holds. We see how people seek relief from the fear of inner fragmentation by handing over their egos to the merged crowd and pay the price of dependency on a charismatic leader who is not task oriented but driven by inner anxiety. Staff and clients in modernising organisations often act like lonely figures in a massed crowd. They resort to desperate measures to seek attention and communicate their need for help and integration. Like the eating disorder patient, some cut themselves to get noticed, some withdraw into autistic bubbles and some legalise all relationships and issue complaints rather than accept a changed reality.

I believe that the experiential world of the neurotic mirrored the pre-1970s organisation and the inner world of the organisation of the 1990s reflects that of the narcissistic and borderline patient. The manic change leader and the narcissistic patient mirror each other and signal a significant shift in the nature and quality of the primary care foundation matrix. Therefore we are in need of different thinking and management methods which take the borderline patient and the disturbed organisational setting as the norm and treat the ordinary neurotic client or manager as the exception. Work with borderline and narcissistic clients implies, for the carer, that self-care becomes the precondition for survival and re-creation. Treatment is only possible when the carer is held and located in a wider matrix, which is dedicated to containment and works towards integration.

What is interesting about the latest primary care reform is that it seems to represent a halfway house between the old and the new organisational paradigms. In putting the onus on local groups to find their own form of institutionalising PCGs, the reform follows the principles of modern organisational thinking which rests on the notions of process, complexity and unpredictability. By launching PCGs within a framework of set targets, a predetermined implementation schedule and review procedures, based on audit and controlling methods, the reform clings to the toolbox approach typical of the old organisational paradigm based on the machine metaphor. I have tried to develop a line of reasoning that clearly leans towards the modern paradigm of an organisation that works more like a chemical reaction than a machine and develops in unpredictable ways. Too much of the thinking that I have encountered among those who try to implement this latest primary care reform is still based on the view of the organisation as an organism that runs like a Newtonian clock and adheres to the Cartesian dichotomy of body and mind. It is the vision that a reform is really predictable and controllable from intent to outcome which hinders, perhaps more than anything, the successful translation of political intent into a reform that reflects the general direction of the goals envisioned, but leaves a genuine space for local innovation.

I want to avoid a denigration of the old ways of organising things and steer clear of an overidealisation of the modern approach, an approach which emphasises visions, missions and evangelical leaders with their followers in reinvented cultural boundaries. The old and the new are not in opposition, they exist in a relationship and derive their meaning through being interdependent and inseparable. Instead of taking sides with either the old or the new, I am adopting a model in which old and new exist in a context and transform each other into new forms of organising and relating within work groups. I see the leader of a work group as one location point in a network of relationships. Although the leader has a special function in guarding the boundary of the group, keeping a focus on the primary task and putting the interests of the group above that of its individual members, he or she is nevertheless not a free agent. Organisational change and its implementation cannot be reduced to the charismatic qualities of the leader and his or her will. The leader is caught in a group matrix that shapes the outcome of a process by involving everyone. Just as the developmental fate of the leader is linked to the capacity for adaptation in the whole work group, so the developmental cycles of organisations can be linked to the transitions from one stage of the life cycle to the next in an individual human being.

Organisations and the human life cycle

Organisational change, such as the setting up of PCGs, is most usefully viewed in terms of the stages and transitions of the human life cycle. In this cycle, the old accomplishments must be relinquished before a person can attach to the next stage of development. Such a transition does not work in the way envisaged by many change leaders in organisations and management books. The human being does not discard the achievements of childhood to adapt to the needs of puberty. We use the need to progress to adolescence and live through its turbulence to regress sufficiently inside to repair the deficits we incurred during earlier transitions. The same happens in organisations and work groups. There is no progress without regression. The choice between relinquishing the old or embracing the new is a false one.

During a change process, the old elements of the self and the old culture of an organisation are reintegrated with the new and form a new self-ideal. This readjusted sense of self is, prior to full acceptance, projected outward and when it is affirmed through other social actors (usually those with authority and in a substitute parent role), it helps us to accept a revised identity in our own eyes – the hardest mirror of them all. With regard to the primary care world I would suggest that an organisational identity suited to the period of the mid-life crisis is called for. In the current context only fundamental questions about why we exist, what we have left to give, what we want to take before we end will help the organisation and the professional within it to move on. What is true for the individual applies to the organisation and the successful primary care reformer will tap the resource of knowledge about transitions in the life cycle locked up in each member of the organisation and work with it rather than against it.

Leadership in a modernised primary care world

The new management culture of devolving responsibility requires a mature and mentally healthy individual. The more open structures in organisations and the push for reaccreditation make it harder to hide incompetence and will increase and extend the forms in which people attempt to hide their weaknesses through some of the psychological defence mechanisms I have already described. Problems in individuals, work groups and organisations derive from disconnectedness and the task of a leader is integration. Leaders can shape the implementation of a reform, but in doing so they will always create unintended side-effects. If they have joined the organisation in order to reform others and avoid changing themselves, they will not be able to integrate the unanticipated outcomes and must resort to ritualised defences. They will not open up a space for learning but, instead, look for faults and people to blame. If, on the other hand, leaders realise that the implementation of the reform has to start with themselves and they can become role models for change, they will be able to shift the mindset of the whole organisation through adjusting their own perspective. Good decision makers will be able to integrate the principles of empathy and authority in their leadership style.

From a psychoanalytic point of view I believe that the most important influence on people in a changing organisational environment is their childhood experience in the family. This shapes people's reactions to the primary care reform more powerfully than the best change management plans and project targets defined by the initiators of the reforms. Father and mother figures in the family tend to show acceptance and approval to the children in different ways. The father figure tends to judge, praise, reject and demand; the mother figure leans towards acceptance and defence, regardless of any merit. The inner child in each of us needs both principles to be upheld and integrated during a transition period. Good organisational leaders will accomplish that task and thereby make an organisation work better as a whole because they keep in touch with the inner child in each PCG member. When the child in the adult is allowed to express itself within a safe group which is led with empathy, then the creative forces can show themselves and the group becomes more than the sum of its parts.

Interdependence in a belonging group

Between the end of the war and the late 1980s the NHS served as a dependable mother and as a belonging group in which our unwanted, split-off, mad and needy parts were contained and held for safekeeping. The trauma of the primary care reforms has been the loss of the idealised organisation, the ideal mother and belonging group. The loss of such an ideal belonging group causes disturbed behaviour patterns in organisations that mirror the bizarre behaviour of withdrawn and inaccessible patients in psychiatry, patients who have withdrawn the truest parts of their core self from social interaction and the accomplishment of the primary task. In such a state of being, their capacity for relatedness and performance meets the carer or manager only in an unrecognisable form. It is like a presenting problem waiting to be recognised, diagnosed, translated and named.

The loss of a belonging group causes the need for primitive forms of mourning in which managers and leaders, like therapists, utilise a technique of tough realism and empathic care whilst avoiding false softness and sentimentality (Tustin, 1986). After the sequence of reforms PCGs will be full of individual members who cannot play an active party in implementing this latest change until they have moved from retreat to anger, to mourning, to reconnection, to dialogue and, finally, to re-creation.

PCGs will have to be able to offer a psychological home, a belonging space, for all those members who have a disturbed relationship with the profession and need to deal with their inner sense of displacement. In this state of displacement, the GPs who have joined a PCG need to relocate their individual professional self within the group and find a role. The whole PCG group, in turn, needs to reposition itself in the wider organisation of the primary care sector and its partners inside and outside the NHS. Perhaps the most important and psychically most difficult task will be the fulfilment of the need of each group and its members to make reparations towards the belonging group of Mother NHS. This means that PCG members need to own their collusion in bringing about the breakdown of the old system of parenting and dependency. When this has been accomplished PCGs and their members can relearn how to live in a state of disillusionment, which is a precondition for making any aspect of this reform work. Only when they start to feel safe enough will GPs accept that they have a need to belong, that they are dependent and that, at the same time, they remain independent and responsible for their own destiny. A healthy belonging group is a precondition for being and staying in the mature and adult position. The sociologist Norbert Elias attempted to overcome the split between the individual and society and he viewed groups as more than the sum of their parts. Individualised solutions and problems set some people up as judge and jury and others as the accused when, in reality, the problem was jointly created and needs jointly to be resolved. Sorting out a malfunctioning GP should involve sorting out the system which has colluded with the creation of this state of dissatisfaction.

Overcoming either/or thinking

Modern organisations will only be able to survive and reinvent themselves if they overcome either/or thinking and adopt instead an as-well-as mindset. Creativity in the individual, the group and the organisation is linked psychically with tension, conflict and uncertainty. It is a force that can never be planned or controlled. According to Elias (1978), thinking, feeling, acting and intent cannot be separately located in an isolated individual but must be seen as processes which involve and reflect social connections and power relations. He called these sets of relationships 'figurations'. The individual thinks and decides, knowingly or unknowingly, in the ebb and flow of being in a relationship and in a group situation – never as an imagined social island. Individuality is only possible in a relationship with other people and is limited by a historical context. Absolute choice to act is, by definition, an illusion, a flight from reality. Psychic independence is always both typical and atypical. We don't possess an 'I' without a 'we'; we cannot be a 'we' without tolerating all the unique 'I's within it. The self defines itself with reference to and in interdependence with the other.

In earlier times human beings were more interested in what they had in common and what their 'we' identity was like. Today, we are more interested in how we differ from others. We want to know what our 'I' is really like. Nevertheless, we can't change our 'we' identities like a new wardrobe each year. Elias wants us to overcome the false opposition between the individual and society, which could be viewed as the conflict between independence and dependence, by viewing all social events as products of relatedness and interdependence. To him, the loss of freedom to act independently entailed in being tied to the group and society was merely the loss of an illusion which had stopped us from holding a sensible and realistic view of life in the first place. The transition in thinking from a focus on individuals as free agents to thinking in relationships, in functions and in a context would, according to Elias, prevent us from arriving at overly idealistic conclusions and thereby make us more pragmatic, democratic and realistic. It would also stop us from splitting the world into goodies and baddies, which leads to authoritarian and punitive forms of behaviour and organisation. If we accept this paradigm, something like reaccreditation will lead to blame and false praise but not to continuous learning, frustration and the capacity to tolerate and master them.

Survival and re-creation in primary care are not linked to predictability and control. Reality, life and organisations are, by definition, unstable and unpredictable. It is therefore important that we leave planning models of organisational change behind and do not just replace it with an evolutionist perspective whereby we simply adapt to a changing environment. We must learn to be sensitive to those changes in the context which we cannot control, accept them, assess the limits of our ability to act independently and then seek to reconstruct ourselves actively in this context of 'bounded chaos'. PCGs will stand or fall by their ability to adopt this mindset.

If the leaders of this latest primary care reform insist on driving the change and bullying the groups into compliance, then the reform will founder and add to the reservoir of disillusionment in primary care. If the leaders of the reform can create favourable conditions within the groups for consultation, support and learning through trial and error, they will give each GP making up these groups the tools for managing the reality of an unknown and uncertain long-term future. Groups and their members who have learnt this lesson can cope with the repeated crises and changes that are now typical of the primary care world. They can individually and collectively hold on to the belief that they can shape the future and that the world will connect with them and make them secure enough to go on learning, surviving and developing. Mental models, sufficient support and a safe belonging group, not managerial toolbags, controlling systems and perfect change management plans, are the key to making the latest primary care reform work.

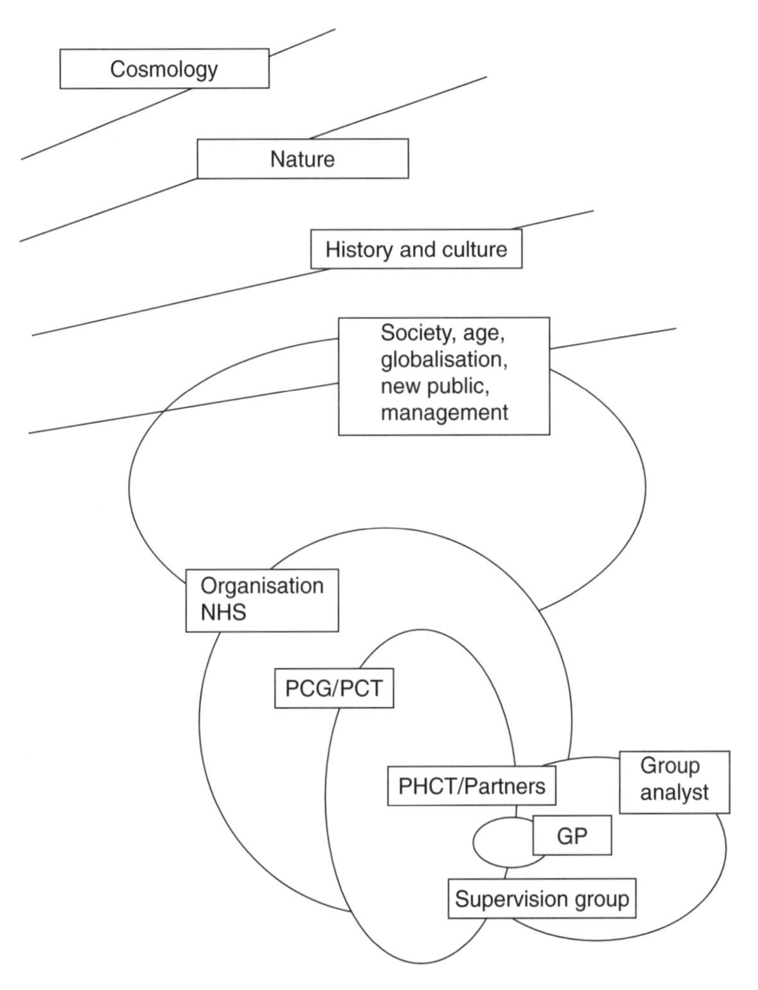

Figure 1.1: The foundation matrix: the context for work, supervision and change in primary care.

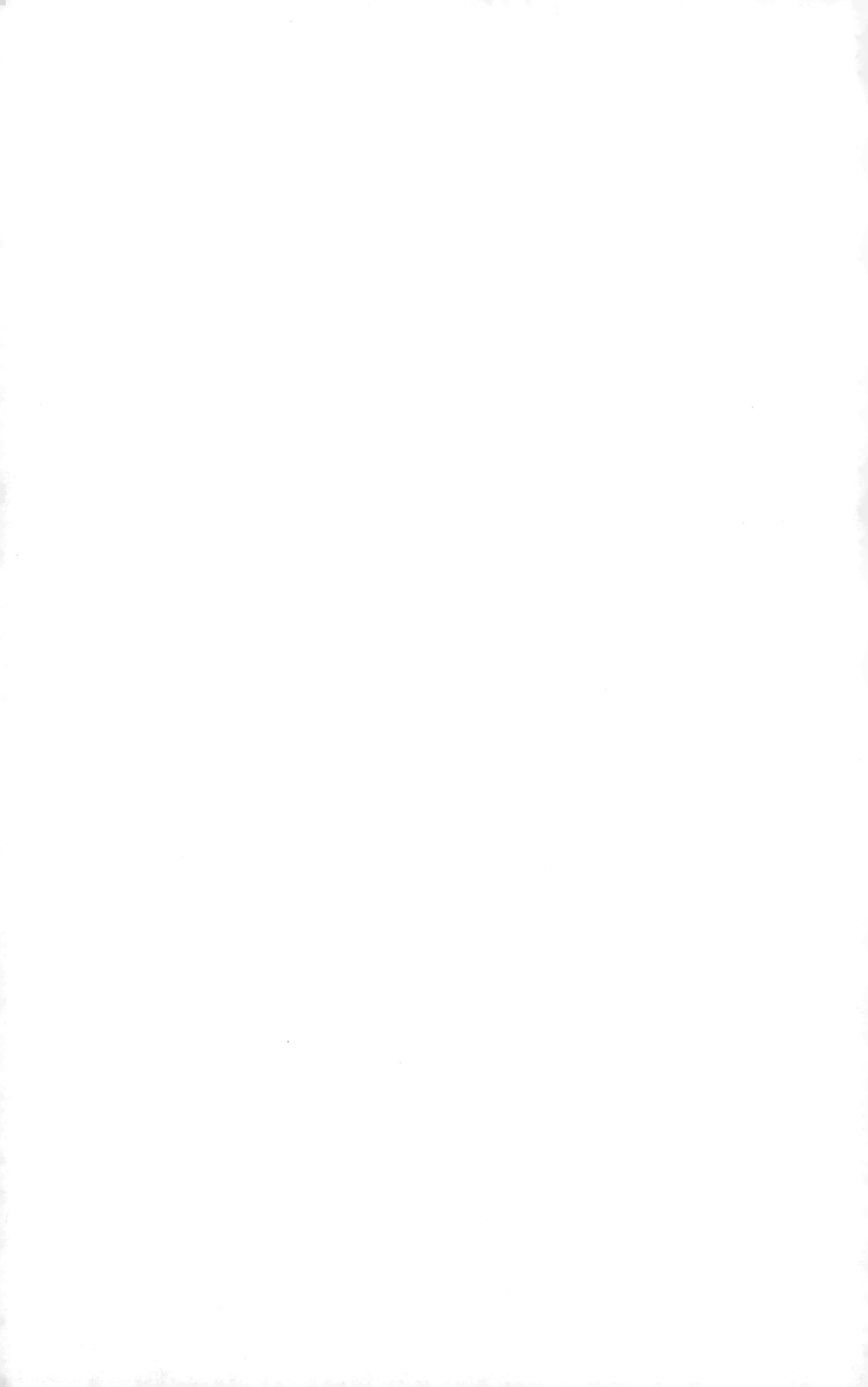

CHAPTER TWO

The group matrix

The acceptance and shaping of change in a partnership

During periods of change in an organisation most of the energy gets projected outward onto the 'persecutors' who drive the unwanted changes or onto the 'scapegoats' who make a last stand of resistance so that a dialogue, mourning and reparation can be avoided.

During a group analytic consultancy intervention I see it as my task to reopen the boundaries between victims and perpetrators, the internal and the external world and between different groups within the organisation. To do that I act as a translator who finds words for the secrets and conflicts which get acted out when an organisation is restructured. Group analysts observe and capture responses to change in metaphors, using words that can contain and hold what is felt and experienced. These verbal interventions, which are called interpretations, act as bridges in a group and make what people experience and feel deep inside exchangeable in a dialogue. Large and small group sessions can help reconnect the flow of communication between different levels of the hierarchy, allow the organisation to let go of policing methods during transition periods and help find ways of adopting a learning model to change management.

This process of widening and deepening the communication, and the search for a shared language within the organisation and between it and the outside world, is not the result of the drive and determination of charismatic change leaders but is accomplished by the group. Resistance to change is only superficially located in the apparently dysfunctional person and is, in reality, a shared experience of the whole group. The group learns through group analysis to relocate the problems of change management in the matrix of the whole organisation. Over time the group develops the 'ego strength' of the individual, the subgroup and the team leader sufficiently to enable each of them to see their interdependence and face up to reality in a mature, autonomous and responsible way.

During the late 1980s, the NHS system was beset by many problems. The search for better solutions continued around issues like access, bed availability, clinical standards, errors and a perceived deterioration in service, particularly in the large conurbations. Against this background the Tomlinson Inquiry was launched to look in detail at the health problems in the London area. Tomlinson called for changes in the organisation, resources and responsibilities of health provision in the primary care sector. The response to the report produced a vision of a 'primary care-led NHS'. Policymakers called for improvements in healthcare and the prevention of disease and for a service that reflected the needs of particular groups and communities. It was envisaged that better relationships between providers and service users should be built up and that health and treatment decisions would be made closer to the patient. The mechanism for delivering these changes was to be the PHCT and consequently GPs were at the interfaces between primary, secondary and tertiary care. Inner-city GPs were put into a special need category and the Tomlinson programme focused on improving premises, community schemes, manpower, clinical services, business and administration methods, computer and information technology and training and teamwork. Despite this extra funding and special attention, many concerns and doubts remained about the new GP Contract and the aims and usefulness of the NHS reforms in primary care.

The 1990 Contract was an integral part of a strategy designed to deliver on *Health of the Nation* targets. London health promotion managers were aware that many GPs recognised the importance of prevention but most saw the new Contract as a form of policing and control, conceived for central political ends and not on the basis of scientific evidence. There was considerable cynicism about purchasers' understanding of realities in primary care amongst fundholders and non-fundholders alike and there were many reasons to think that PHCTs felt undervalued and simply not listened to at any level.

Funding was made available for a consultancy-cum-research intervention which tried to understand the concerns of the professionals in PHCTs and develop ways of working with the 1993 Contract so that the change grew out of their experience and helped them work in a less stressful way (Binney *et al.*, 1995). The most important reason for calling in consultants (Gerhard Wilke and George Binney) was to listen to the experiences of a PHCT and move nearer to understanding how key players tried to translate policy intentions into healthcare or health promotion practice and learn how to move the reform on. As consultants, we wanted to offer an alternative to telling doctors what to comply with. We wanted to enter the primary care world like social anthropologists and learn, through participant observation and in-depth interviews, how to illuminate the difficulties, as well as the good qualities, of the primary care culture. We needed to know more about the way the new GP Contract was being accepted and how it was being modified and shaped in practice before making any recommendations about how to move the reform process on. We hoped that through an essentially qualitative research method, firm results would identify common ground and bring some insight to the situation that a mere recitation of descriptive statistics could hardly do.

We had a strong hunch that we were dealing with powerful feelings. We expected that this work, conducted within a limited budget, would experiment with different perspectives but would not iron out every problem encountered. We hoped that the results would be trusted in themselves without being discounted as unrepresentative, invalid or unworthy of generalisation. Finally, we hoped that the outcome might help to give relevant support to a PHCT and benefit patients.

The consultancy-cum-research approach was built on four connected elements:

- working with an advisory group composed of a cross-section of key players – a university research group, managers from regions and FHSAs, a GP and a practice manager – which defined terms of reference for the project and guided and supported its implementation

- interviewing a range of professionals involved in the field to identify key issues affecting health promotion in primary care
- working with two practices to address the issues which they saw as important and explore them in a practical way
- offering the lessons from work with the two practices to others (PHCTs, managers, academics and policymakers) in discussion and via publications.

We went beyond simply researching what exists and explored what could be different: how individual practices, with outside support, could begin to shape change. We believed that the strength of this consultancy-cum-research approach lies in the fact that it moves the participants from being passive objects for research into the role of active co-researcher and change agent. The consultancy process gets away from the split between experts and infantilised objects of change management and becomes a joint search for learning, knowledge and solutions. The exchange of experience involved in the process produces a degree of openness and trust that makes it easier to accept and implement the changes identified. Change works best if not just the professional in role but the whole person engages in the process.

Two practices met with us about eight times and worked through their recent experiences of primary care reform. Through a dialogue at both the task and emotional levels, participants moved from an unconscious to a more conscious understanding of how they relate to each other, their work and the implementation of the GP Contract and health promotion in primary care.

Paradoxical effect of the NHS reforms

The 1990 and 1993 GP Contracts imposed an additional burden on primary care teams without achieving the objective of markedly increasing the amount of effective health promotion work in primary care. The data collection process required by the Contracts was generally seen as something needed to feed the bureaucracy of health and not contributing to real health promotion. Among many GPs, community nurses, health visitors and also managers, we met a feeling of frustration and powerlessness, of having made substantial efforts to change the behaviour of patients but with few clear results.

During the early 1990s individuals at all levels in the system felt that they were caught up in a pattern of endless new initiatives, poorly conceived and executed. As one initiative failed to deliver the promised results, managers and health politicians responded by trying harder, instituting yet more initiatives and reorganisations which in their turn disappointed. At each level in the system the picture of frustration and exhaustion seemed to repeat itself. NHS managers at regional level felt imposed upon by the NHS HQ and frustrated because they could not obtain the results they needed from FHSAs. Managers in FHSAs felt imposed upon by Region and anxious because primary care teams did not respond as they wanted. Doctors were irked by the requirements coming from managers and were obliged to impose on their staff things that they found distasteful. Nurses, practice managers and receptionists felt that they were not listened to by doctors. As a therapist I felt that if the NHS were a patient, I would have said that it was suffering a manic depressive breakdown.

Communications between different parts of the system were poor and there was frequently a lack of trust and an inability to understand the perspective of others. The changes of the early 1990s appeared overwhelming to the PHCT members and, from a psychoanalytic point of view, the team and its individual members appeared as a helpless and dependent baby. Metaphorically speaking, the PHCT baby was stuck in a relationship with an NHS parent who had moved from being nurturing and attuned to the needs of the baby into a malignant and cannibalistic position. The new regime (environmental mother) was experienced as consuming the true self (professional self-ideal) and the baby was required to present a false self in order to comply with the mother's neurotic needs (e.g. monitoring system). The baby began to imagine that any expression of its own desires would hasten the mother's imminent death. To prevent such a trauma the baby started to comply.

At an unconscious level the group dynamic within a PHCT was, at that time, dominated by the fear of losing the NHS and one's own livelihood and change was experienced as a form of persecution, a threat of annihilation. Reality seemed very difficult to bear and the vulnerable PHCTs had withdrawn into an imaginary world and looked for safety in defensive manoeuvres or in Utopian visions of a lost paradise. People had regressed from being conscious of their own actions to acting out their helplessness and their need for safety. They heard the demand to grow up but they felt infantilised. Those who tried to manage the change process felt as if they were in charge of a group of resentful, delinquent children who should know better and needed to be closely monitored because they evidently did not know how to behave and be good girls and boys. A mutually collusive system of manic-depressive ways of relating was set up between the different key players. Healthy alliances, which were meant to be set up and develop within and beyond the team, were sabotaged.

The PHCTs in reaction: a sense of powerlessness

The difficulties with health promotion were closely related to problems of leadership and management. There was a lack of clear direction and priorities. Many staff were not sure what importance to attach to health promotion or which areas to focus on. There was a sense of powerlessness, and energy went into pushing the responsibility for health promotion on to others or back up the line (the government, schools, industry, Social Services) rather than looking at what primary care teams could do, had done and might want to do. Team members inhabited a mythical past and future and retreated from the reality of the here and now. There was a reluctance to confront openly problems such as difficulties with poorly performing staff. Due to fear of non-compliance, it was also difficult to acknowledge publicly the very different perspectives of health promotion that existed. The doctors often abdicated elements of their responsibility for leadership and management and transferred (both practically and psychologically) an overwhelming burden on to the practice manager and the receptionists.

Unintended consequences of the reforms had displaced the intended outcomes. With imposed change the pressure on the developing PHCT to operate in the adult mode had produced more regression into childish forms of behaviour rather than greater autonomy. The message to be adult was heard at an unconscious level as: My true professional self is not good enough, I have to present a false self to make the parent think that I am good. My safety, identity and sense of belonging depend on conforming and I must turn the way I feel, the way I think and my experience into a secret. Most of all, I must hide the fact that I make mistakes and that I have weaknesses. Families with secrets distort relationships and stunt growth and development. Similar relationships had developed between a PHCT and other parts of the NHS system when health promotion statistics produced and presented for evaluation then became the basis on which the team was resourced by the system. The family began to live the myth it had created and could no longer relate adequately to the truth, that the feedback to the system had been doctored to get the system off the team's back. The PHCT, trapped in this charade, became unable to own its mistakes and weaknesses and hence incapable of learning from experience. Patterns of relationships, methods of communication and getting the work done took on the feel of a repetition compulsion.

PHCT defences

The PHCT I worked with preferred the compliant child position to that of the autonomous adult. It was better to be monitored, told what to do and present false statistics than to lose the NHS as a mother and be left with rivalrous peers. Facing the peer group involved choosing the first amongst equals to lead the partnership. This position drained the PHCT members of their creative energy and reinforced their tendency to respond defensively to any message from the outside world. The organisational parents (managers/reformers/partners) needed to find a way of making it safe for team members to give up their need to be dependent and rediscover that their own experience of life had taught them that they could change, and needed to. Making the link between life experience and the need for change enabled team members to move on.

This is easier than it sounds because the problems of practice management are mitigated by the very high levels of personal commitment demonstrated by primary care professionals, managers and staff and the motivation they derive from direct patient contact and care. I found that, given some support to confront uncomfortable issues, there was a high degree of openness and willingness to consider new ways of working. The change potential within a PHCT can be tapped if managers and change leaders have the courage to develop relationships based on trust and avoid imposing change in such a way that the objects of their reforms are cast in the role of naughty children. This change in attitude at the leadership level would enable denigratory relationships to be transformed into working alliances and remove the fear that prevents real change from taking root.

The managerial and adviser level

In the 1990s, managers at all levels needed to be enabled to slow down and listen more. Paradoxically, those who tried less hard achieved more. There were many people within primary care wanting to undertake effective health promotion who needed encouragement and support. Many nurses I interviewed saw health promotion as an opportunity to broaden their role and gain more recognition. Many individual doctors were ideologically happy to make a contribution to health promotion, although generally as a very subsidiary part of their jobs. The capacity to cope would have increased after the 1990 and 1993 Contracts if those concerned with improving the system had placed less emphasis on the 'policing' aspect of monitoring and evaluation and instead engaged with PHCTs in a process designed to examine the results openly and critically.

There was a need for those delivering the reforms in practice to move away from generalised statements that 'Health promotion is a good thing' to a critical examination of what primary care teams could realistically and most effectively contribute. There needed to be more clearly defined limits to what could be done by a PHCT. The absence of clear boundaries to the reform task led to the construction of omnipotent change fantasies designed to deny that death and illness, social norms and resistance to them were part of normal life. The *Health of the Nation* documents and the evangelists who acted as primary care advisers were in danger of doing this because they had a naive view of how PHCTs and patients could be re-educated.

As a coach and trainer, I have learnt that new knowledge is not necessarily received well by workshop participants. Many learners who seek change experience the diet they are given by reformers and educators as an attack on their fragile identity. Instead of extending their horizon, absorbing new ways of thinking, they end up having an identity crisis and start acting like a bulimic. They manically binge on the change 'food' and then vomit it out in secret, instead of internalising it and holding on to the nourishment contained in the 'food for thought'. Health managers and PHCT members applied for jobs as primary care advisers, promised the earth in their job interviews, and then found themselves resorting to re-education techniques which were manipulative and authoritarian. Instead of coming nearer each other during local organising team (LOT) workshops and creating a real working alliance, the gap between PHCT members and health authority change leaders widened.

Change would have been accepted more easily if planners and managers had recognised the unknown as a normal part of the implementation process. If the idea of uncertain, unpredictable outcomes was really integrated into the planning process, it would become safer to trust, make mistakes, take risks and let go of fear. Loss can only be faced in the mature position if change leaders are accepting of the regressive side of human nature. By acknowledging the need for resistance to change and the anger against the initiators and by having the inner fear of a significant loss named, the change leader creates a space in a group to let go, move on and embrace the new. Instead of labelling critics as resisters of change and backward looking, policymakers, managers and team leaders should seek to understand the factors that underlie the critics' scepticism: the increased pressure primary care workers experience when they are asked to deliver the normal service whilst simultaneously changing patient behaviour. Audit should function to encourage genuine efforts to understand what has happened in practice. It should not be a cold statistical exercise but involve an exchange of experiences in order to learn from success and failure and shape change in the light of such reflections. Audits should not just be a methodology for enforcing budgetary and professional discipline and dividing GPs into black and white sheep.

The PHCT level

PHCTs could have done much to help themselves in the early 1990s. They could have started to identify the areas where they had a chance to shape their own futures. For this to happen, partners within practices would have had to talk to each other more frankly than they did. Only through real dialogue, including conflict about substantial issues, could they have taken more collective responsibility for development and change. In many cases the opportunity was missed because it was preferable to stay in the victim position and cry for help by resisting the advances of the reforming authorities. Unconsciously, GPs were asking the system to recognise the need for boundaries, limits and a slower speed of change. This indicates to me that many doctors were sufficiently traumatised by the reforms to be unable to express their need for support in words or negotiate their way forward. They could only communicate their distress to the health authority by rituals of non-compliance and it is the change leaders who recognised this form of resistance as a communication and not an act of aggression who were able to help such doctors embrace the new order.

The sheer volume and unrelenting pressure of reform seems to have come up against the limited capacity of individuals and groups to internalise and integrate the change. After many years of being left alone, adopting new working practices was not simply a matter of adding a new habit to an existing routine. The impact of change went much deeper as each adjustment amounted to a loss and an attendant mourning process was required. If teams had been given more time and space to mourn, their capacity to accept and shape change would have developed. It is not anger and resentment but sadness that is the precondition for repairing the loss and integrating the new. The route to re-creation in primary care is through survival and mourning. Any change scheme that tries to avoid these regressive phases and wants to move into the 'New Jerusalem' of primary care without pain and chaos will end up in false compliance. Groups within the organisation need to stop retreating into a defensive stance and maintain and develop good external relations before new forms of organisation can take hold. Only then can the key players in an organisation develop the capacity to say yes and no appropriately to other unidisciplinary groups and the existing hierarchy demanding change.

The world of one partnership

The Jocelyn Chamberlain Unit at St George's Medical School in London conducted a research-cum-consultancy project to find ways in which PHCTs could be helped to move away from rejecting change and find their own ways of shaping the future of their partnerships. The research hypothesis was that a team could find and adopt change more easily if the incoming agent of change did not predefine the direction and content. I wanted to test the idea that a negotiated entry into the practice, a short research phase and a limited number of open group sessions could generate more improvements in the delivery of the service than the best worked-out change programme imposed from outside. A member of a local medical committee (LMC) agreed to recommend participation in the project.

I was invited to the next partner meeting and during this discussion it emerged that the 1990 Contract had unsettled the practice and had made some partners willing to call in outsiders to do some work on the team and communication systems. It also became clear that other partners were not keen on opening what was described as Pandora's box. After some discussion of the fears that people had about a process of open and honest talking, the partner group agreed to participate in the project. It was agreed that the whole PHCT should be involved in the background research and interviews but the facilitated group sessions would only include the partners and the practice manager.

What the in-depth interviews revealed

I interviewed for two days after having agreed dates and delegating the task of compiling a batting order to the practice manager. She had decided that it would be best to see as many people as possible in order to minimise feelings of being left out. I saw some people individually and others in pairs or even as small focus groups. It had been agreed that open questions would be asked to establish the real issues. I also wanted to use the research phase to begin helping the group to take responsibility for finding some solutions to the problems they identified. I felt it necessary to remain task focused enough to allow the 'commissioners' of the project to gain an insight into the interplay between health promotion and general practice management. On this basis I agreed to ask: What is working for you in this practice, what is not working for you in this practice, what are the issues for you around health promotion, what are the issues for you around the management of the PHCT and what solutions do you have?

The issues that emerged during the interviews were connected by some overarching themes. First, communication and the need to exchange ideas and feelings in a more frank way so that people could own their collective and individual responsibilities more effectively. Second, the theme of leadership and decision making and the clarification of responsibilities. Third, the issue of strategy and the desire for clear direction and a sense of priorities for the practice. Finally, I met with a widespread feeling that the team was in the grip of a paralysing non-confrontational culture that made it difficult to adjust working practices and shape the changes which the PHCT was expected to implement. In what follows I introduce 'dramatis personae' into the text – all exist but their names have been changed to preserve anonymity. During the interview phase and in the two group sessions with the whole PHCT on the research-cum-consultancy process, I talked to a cross-section of the team and the names reflect a range of roles and functions. In the detailed accounts of the small group sessions only the partners and the practice manager were present.

Communication

As a supplementary question I had asked Anna whether there were any splits, apart from the one between the partners and the other staff in the practice. She revealed that there was a divide between part-time and full-time staff and between the early and late shift. Communicating across the barriers was difficult and she found herself in a position where she had almost been at the practice longest but felt treated as if she were the most junior and recent arrival. Consequently, it was difficult to speak in meetings: 'I withdraw and talk to my husband in private. He does the same, especially when he has taken a lot of the management issues upon himself and then gets too little thanks in return.'

Lucille, one of the nurses, compared the good old days, when there were three partners and an atmosphere of openness, trust, initiative and self-management, with the new situation when things were dominated by group processes, systems, structures and targets. She used to be clear about her role and responsibilities.

Now she felt that she did what she was told but didn't know what the limits of her responsibilities were supposed to be. Things were now done as a favour between the different professionals. She talked of the need to spell out who was in charge and who could be asked to take on extra tasks. The team had been enlarged and there was more pressure. Under stress, unkind remarks were overinterpreted and there was no place for the outspoken person. People very quickly sulked and hit back with sarcasm. This then influenced how the workload was allocated: some were protected, some got punished. She highlighted the need to get away from being a happy crew to being a caring and honest crew.

Leadership and decision making

John (one of the partners) had been my link person and it was therefore not really surprising to find him flagging up the decision-making and leadership issue. He described himself as being in the initiator, inventor and enforcer role. It became apparent in the interview that holding power and responsibility was difficult for him. He talked about feeling exposed and not being supported enough by the partners. Secretly, he feared that the other partners experienced him as too forceful and they harboured resentment against him. He wondered whether there was a power split within the partner group, with the men holding the power of speech and the women the power of silence. For a leader, he appeared to give himself too hard a time over the issue of needing to be fair and ensuring that everyone's voice was heard. These symptoms of mistrust made me feel that he was not speaking for himself but lending a voice to the value system of the group. He seemed to be looking to the consultancy process to give him legitimacy as a leader and justify his bid to have management responsibilities in the practice clarified. He wanted to shift the partner group from only saving the patients to learning that doctors have to manage staff and staff must learn to manage the patients and the partners. To put it another way, he was looking to move from a dependency mode within the practice to a better network of relationships in which it was possible to take on responsibility and leadership without feeling defensive and guilty.

I saw Sam and Janet together. Both had worked as receptionists in the practice for many years and regarded themselves as experts on the old and new ways. They were at the sharp end of mediating between patient and doctor and between the demand for service outstripping the supply of care. The conflict which ruled their lives was that between the number of appointments in the book and the availability of doctors. They gave me the sense that a lot of problems would be solved if only the doctors were more available inside the practice and would stop playing about outside.

> We know these doctors. What is agreed this week is different next week. Doctors vary a lot: some we can cajole to fit the extra person in, others don't budge. Mind you, patients now fit the doctor into their appointment calendar. It's the kids to school first, then the hairdresser and then us. The patients decide who needs to be seen, we don't. They complain otherwise or, when a doctor has refused to see them, they ask for one who will. In the old days patients had respect for the doctors and for us. Many of them don't now.

In other words, decisions were made by those who shouted loudest at the counter or over the phone. It is interesting that this mirrors one of the comments made by a partner, who pointed out that the workload was allocated in order to pacify the complainers and objectors among the staff and in the partner group.

Another theme of this culture of making decisions by default emerged in two separate interviews with nurses in the team. Jennifer told me what it felt like to be scapegoated and Evelyn what it was like to have to work with the scapegoat. The scapegoat was asking me why no one recognised her strengths and worked to them. Her colleague was asking why nobody sorted out the behaviour of her deviant colleague. When I probed a bit deeper I found that at the core of the conflict around decision making there was an inability to let go of the past and a lack of confidence in facing the here and now in a grown-up way. Elizabeth, a third nurse, pointed out that this was a delightful team to be in, especially the nurses group, except for the inclusion of one person who was a spoiler.

Teams like locating their problems in one person because then that person can be labelled as morally deficient and the other members of the group look healthy and perfect in comparison. The alternative is more difficult to face as it would involve all team members recognising how the scapegoat's behaviour is really only an exaggerated version of everyone's flawed behaviour. As Elizabeth put it:

> I don't know how one worker can be allowed to take so many liberties without being taken on and controlled. We have all tried to please her but that seems to make it worse. Sometimes when I was strict it seemed to improve things, one of the partners has got to act as an authority figure. The younger doctors find that difficult. The patients don't help because they still hanker after the older doctors who have retired. So, the good doctors have gone and the ones here don't really want to sort things out.

Again, it was striking that this seemed to be a re-enactment within the system of the stuck parts in the relationship between the receptionists, doctors and patients. It was the tail wagging the dog. It was the 'naughty child' in the family acting out what everyone secretly wished for: to be able to get away with not complying with the new and much tighter system of control.

Strategy and direction

Two of the partners, Stephen and John, wanted this topic to be dealt with and stressed the need to get every partner to outline their wishes and ideas. They saw this as the key to changing the decision-making process in the practice and setting new priorities. They wanted to shape the change from within the practice rather than simply react to agendas set by outside agencies.

Anna made the link between strategy and poor communication when she pointed out that one of the blockages was the degree of disillusionment felt because the practice had lost the older, senior partner and with him a sense of direction.

> Not all partners have the same aim and the practice

> doesn't know where it is going. Partners all inhabit their own worlds. This is normal but in times of great change we need to work together, but not every partner is trusted equally and can be relied upon to work to the same standard. If the one or two people who carry a lot of the management burden left tomorrow, there would be chaos. A lot of things are kept private which should be discussed professionally and openly. We struggle with being different, with facing up to our real strengths.

It sounded a bit like a family in mourning, where issues of inheritance and succession have not yet been settled and those affected are still preoccupied with the feelings appropriate to bereavement. Feelings of disorientation and resentment at the unfairness of the loss predominated. The dead father was idealised rather than replaced. This happens because people would rather keep a ghost alive and find fault with each other than face up to looking at the potential for leadership in the successors and sorting out who deserves to lead and who doesn't.

At a deeper level the matrix of this PHCT was paralysed by the mixed messages from the foundation matrix of the health authority and society. The ideology of the multidisciplinary team follows the logic of management fashion and wants to make the work group flatter, less hierarchical and more inclusive. The PHCT needed clarification of the hierarchy after the retirement of the senior partner. It was obvious to me that we needed to face the selection of one clearly identifiable leader at the expense of other contenders. The failure to mourn resulted in a retreat into psychologically defensive positions within the work group. In the face of the task of implementing major changes, some members had become overdependent on the imagined or actual leader(s), others split into subgroups which became more inward looking and started to play territorial demarcation games and yet others started to fight and flee from the consequences of their aggression. The common ground for the team members became the increased need to keep reality at bay. The energy went into the construction of an exceedingly polite culture of communication in which only safe topics were named and anything threatening was avoided.

Culture of the practice

Stephen appeared like a man who had been sitting on things for a long time. 'We have a culture of appeasement,' he blurted out at the start of the interview and then went on to say that partners fitted in well and shared ideas about primary care but that they had very different ideas about how to work things out in practice. In over five years of change there had not been a major dispute and everybody was busy shying away from conflict. It was difficult to get to a point where strategic issues for the practice could really be discussed and fundamental decisions were made by default. When I asked a follow-up question about the difficulties associated with conflict, he said that there were three levels at work: first, the values people held; second, the personalities involved; and third, the systems set up to manage the practice.

> We are a religious practice and hold strong Samaritan beliefs and yet we run a business. There is therefore a split. When we all meet we keep to the agenda and are very polite to each other. Some don't want to face the business issues. John is left with them. When we meet in private, at our prayer meeting, quite different agendas emerge, we then talk about stress, how difficult it all is, the complaints we get, how overwhelmed we feel by the changes and our uncertainty about where we go next.

When I asked where his resentment goes, he answered that he, like everyone else, had to let it out elsewhere.

> I do get angry inside and I do feel very resentful sometimes. But those who make least fuss get more loaded up, like a workhorse. Those partners who make more fuss get relieved because the staff react by shifting their work elsewhere. This is the real problem with our culture, the workload and responsibilities are almost private matters. It would help if we could start to talk more openly about what we actually do and assess the total workload realistically. We are obsessive about having the same number of appointments but don't give

the person in charge of the computers or the finances enough time and space to take on these responsibilities properly. The same is true of new ideas, I can throw in ideas when changes come but I am not so good at seeing them implemented. We are not open enough to connect the people with ideas and those who can see things through. Often it gets left to the practice manager to implement the ideas, but that person is part of the appeasement process.

Health promotion and the GP Contract

'Health promotion, as part of the Contract, has made us think about using the computer as a tool in preventative medicine, but I must say that staff are better at entering data than partners,' said Stephen, when I asked him about health promotion (HP). This answer illustrated a general point about this part of the interviews, that the answers reflected the professional role or the special interest of the interviewee. It was only John who, in his capacity as a LMC representative, adopted both a practice-specific and a wider systemic view. He said that the practice had embraced the HP part of the GP Contract without much difficulty. It was also true that GPs were resentful and cynical because they saw no proof that there would be good outcomes, that health checks could be shown to be of real benefit and that the real purpose was not rooted in political dogma. He was resentful because he had to do more work for the same money and HP had created additional work for the PHCT and increased expenditure for the NHS. 'If you look for high blood pressure you'll find it and will have to prescribe medication and make referrals to consultants.' The central problem, as he saw it, was that everyone in the PHCT and in the FHSA doubted the sincerity of the reforms and suspected hidden government agendas. The whole thing was seen as a political ploy designed to prove the government right at the doctors' expense.

At the practice level he said that some GPs hated HP and others liked it. Everyone was involved at a basic level but the enthusiasts took the lead and ran the clinics. The guiding principle was to devolve clinical responsibility to the nurses. The major problem for the nurses was the mix of full-time and part-time employees and the issue of co-operation between them. Just as the partners had a leadership problem, so did the nurses. It surfaced around HP because it confronted them with the changes they could make by taking on more responsibility and redefining the way they related to patients and doctors. I couldn't resist pointing out that the focal conflicts among the senior staff were usually mirrored at a lower level in the organisation in some way. As far as healthy alliances go, a partner pointed out that the practice had minimal interaction with the FHSA and members of the PHCT resented facilitators and would rather see the money spent on care and treatment.

The problem of feeling only partly connected to the whole NHS system was the strongest theme in my interview with June, one of three health visitors at the practice.

> We are paralysed by being pig in the middle. There is a 'them and us' situation. We belong to the trust, they belong to the practice. The doctors try to include us but we sense that we are not 100% part of the place. It wouldn't occur to the practice to really inform and consult us when they change their systems. So we live in between and belong to neither, we liaise as separate professionals but don't really come together. The links are determined by the tasks, not by what we have agreed together and want to achieve.

Rachel was a doctor who saw the point of a new GP Contract. The interview with her was wide-ranging and demonstrated that the themes which I have flagged up in this chapter cannot really be separated out and together they reflect the whole culture of the primary care sector. She pointed out that:

> One cannot separate practice management and health promotion. Health promotion is about the whole person and the prevention of disease and good management is about the whole team and the prevention of crises and complaints. We must pick things up early enough. We do quite well but the issue is that we could, and need to, do better in the face of change. The biggest problem is that some partners refer to the clinics we run and others don't; some want a shift from treatment to the clinics and others don't. The other big blocks are: computerisation, the

> telephonists and receptionists. The old hands in the practice don't recognise HP as important and we end up with a split between the doctors who want to do real medicine and those who don't. All this gets translated into the appointment system and makes for an attitude problem amongst staff, some of whom end up being obstructive and trying to score points around the issue of booking appointments for the HP clinics.

When I asked her for a way forward, it emerged that the biggest block was the fact that the partners were afraid of confrontation and decision making. This prevented them from setting priorities, providing leadership to the staff and supporting each other in finding an appropriate management role within the practice. I asked her who she identified as the actual or potential leader and she mentioned two of the partners but excluded herself. I pointed this out and suggested that it was perhaps a way of linking the leadership and attitude problem in a different way. If every partner could start to own the leader in themselves and if every other member of the PHCT started to think about being responsible for the whole team, the whole workload and not just their own specialist area could be managed in a less stressful way.

Change in the group, through the group, with the group

Partner and practice manager only groups

Group 1

At the end of the interviewing process I drew up a short report which outlined the strengths and weaknesses of the practice. The report was circulated and the first group session was dominated by giving feedback and offering group members a space in which to reflect on and respond to what I had found. After I had given a verbal version of the report I simply asked what their impressions were when they read the report and which themes they would like to pick up and sort out. Stephen was anxious to speak and grabbed the space. His response was: 'The picture is accurate. I recognise our central problems. We avoid confrontation and we fear the perceived consequences. We are too cautious, and avoid asking how we can get there'.

I asked where and when.

> Well, around meetings. You highlight that our informal gatherings meet some important needs, but that we need help with how we negotiate change. Perhaps we could exchange our particular agendas and find out the common ground and the differences we have. I would like to start to identify obstacles to being more open with one another in meetings.

At this point the latecomers arrived and Stephen broke off and filled them in on what had happened so far. He was clearly irritated about the lateness but came across as being at great pains not to offend anyone and gave a fair summary of events so far. What he had really wanted to do was to finish his important story. Now it had been interrupted. The culture had been restored. The communication flow leading to greater intimacy had been broken. He finished very abruptly: 'I have a picture of everyone's agenda in my head but we never discuss the important items on that agenda'.

Rachel then spoke:

> Communication is a problem. The statements about change reminded me of recent events in my own life, like moving house and all the disruption that caused. I have problems with a life-long aversion to conflict. I feel that the eloquent people in this team get heard in meetings, whereas I get uptight before meetings and need courage to speak. The other problem about communication is that people are not clear about who reports to whom. The lines are blurred. The staff should report to the practice manager but some have a preferred relationship with a particular doctor and it becomes difficult to refer patients back when you think inappropriate appointments have been made. Some staff play one doctor off against another and we need to find a way of addressing some of these issues more consistently through a staff meeting.

Wendy, the practice manager, interrupted at this point and said that some of this was rubbish. She seemed threatened by what was coming up in this unfamiliar kind of meeting with no fixed agenda and with people sitting in a circle and spending 90 minutes together.

Rachel was not deterred and continued, 'I wish we could learn to be better personnel managers, I want to clarify roles and delegate better'.

I asked who should take this on. 'Hilda, because she has been here the longest, and me, as I feel very strongly about it.'

Thomas then took his turn and said:

> We need to talk about another important person in our practice. It is God. God is more taboo than sex or other subjects, except that our evangelical commitments get into everything. Our priority is to build good healing relationships, they are the key to everything, this includes the relationship to God. It is that which prevents me from embracing the new NHS and I feel safe in here but unsafe out there. Leadership is different for us; it is not about assertion, it is about self-sacrifice.

When he was asked what he wished to accomplish in this group, he answered that he wanted to understand better how people tick. What prevented him saying what he wanted of the partners was that he felt indebted to them and therefore didn't think he could make more demands. I asked him what else he could give to the practice. He answered that he could be the lead person on audits.

Hilda offered her view that the report was broadly accurate and that she agreed with Rachel that personnel management was the priority for her. She also felt that she ended up dealing with most of these matters because she was perceived as the most senior person. It was pointed out to her that this might be because she managed to stay aloof and did not get overinvolved. 'That is how it should be,' she answered. Paula took over this theme and revealed that she had no problem with staying detached but found it difficult to assert herself. Conflict was something abhorrent and therefore she too found it difficult to crystallise what she wanted. For her, the consultancy should be about exploring the rift between the old and the new guard and finding out what partners wanted beyond being a good doctor. The other theme for her was a reduction in the workload and the fact that there was perhaps too much altruism in the practice.

From a consultant's point of view, the group was working very hard now and it was noticeable that the practice manager and the latecomers had not spoken. The group would end without a clear contribution from the practice manager, communicating to us the fact that she was ambivalent about her membership of the partner group. This made me question whether she had a very clear place and role in the decision-making process itself. It was noticeable in this context that she, unlike the partners, wore the staff uniform.

The latecomers were the last to reflect on the report. John started with his wishes for the group sessions. He wanted to improve working relationships and relate more honestly. He wanted it recognised that there were real differences of opinion and interest among the partners. He saw the group as being preoccupied with what the world of primary care should be like rather than how it was. This had become clear to him during the discussion about fundholding, when he had been the only partner wanting to adopt this model. He thought people felt that the partners believed that non-fundholding meant more clinical commitment and less time spent on management, adding up to better patient care. I pointed out that his statements were connected with some of the issues brought up by Thomas. They both agreed that the partners' ethical beliefs had made it more difficult to adopt the fundholding option. John thought there was no point in reopening the fundholding issue and that he would find it more useful to concentrate on the management of staff in the group sessions.

Anna defended the private prayer meetings which some partners came to and that had become a focus for sharing the stress caused by life in the practice. She pointed out that even these more intimate meetings still did not go deep enough for her and that she was looking to the consultant to help the partners become 'more real with each other'.

> I want us to start touching the real issues and to feel under less pressure to fit in all the time. We do not value each other enough, I certainly don't feel valued as a full doctor. The on-call system is the main mechanism for

> exclusion and inclusion in the practice and we need to look at that.

At this point I said that it was time to stop but Hilda and Rachel had the last word by expressing their regret that the prayer meetings had not been there for everyone. From this, I knew that the group looked for integration and a common ground whilst retaining a sense of difference.

Group 2

The practice manager was on holiday and John and Anna were late again. I started the group off by asking what people had taken away the last time and what they were bringing this time. Paula, who had always been quiet before, started off by saying that she had pondered on why life was so hectic and how it could be managed better. It was difficult for her to manage her time, she felt guilty a lot of the time and felt very stressed in relation to parts of health promotion where she took the lead in the practice. She was asked what the main stress factors were and she replied that writing the protocol was very stressful, filling in the form was easy but doing the audit was causing anxiety as it seemed so pointless. When asked how she managed to take the audit seriously when she didn't believe in its validity, she answered:

> We are involved in a cynical data collection exercise or have made it so. The problem is how to get 15% growth and show it. We don't really have the time to achieve this in reality, we can't offer the patients anything new so it boils down to getting colleagues to record information on the computer to get the figures to match up.

Stephen, who was the computer expert in the practice, added: 'It is useful to have a full picture but the financial incentives work against us doing it properly. What is required is a step-by-step approach to the whole thing and we should get money for it at each stage'. Several people then shared their general cynicism about government intent.

I asked whether there was any real energy for health promotion anywhere in the practice. A lively discussion ensued from which the following points emerged: there was an overcrowded agenda already; health promotion got marginalised; and no one sensed that there was real corporate ownership of health promotion within the practice or within the regional system, as there were other, more important, agendas around all the time. Someone then said:

> We have had one project here which interested everybody and energised those involved. The reason for this was that we all saw the point of it and we all linked up effectively. The problem is that most models of intervention are out of sync with the latest research and practice, and what we get under the present arrangements are the worried-well and what we don't get are those groups who we didn't get in the old days either. The biggest issue is physical exercise and there are no targets set in this area.

The group was beginning to move into the position of the helpless victim again. In response, I asked how any of this linked in with the people in this group. John took this up:

> We do have an attitude problem linked to this because we hold out against fundholding and, consequently, avoid the question of where we are going. We avoid finding out how we want to project ourselves. Do we want to be Luddites? Do we want to be a serious opposition, is anyone positively wanting to embrace some of the changes?

The group took this up at the level of general practice philosophy and communication, avoiding the more difficult questions to do with money and business. People found common ground in saying that they perceived the reallocation of some chronic disease treatment from secondary to primary care as valuable and that they also broadly embraced the division which was emerging in the system, with specialists placed in hospital settings and generalists in primary care.

The group then started to explore some of the communication gaps that everyone was aware of and wanted something done about.

> We need to find a way of sharing our approaches to clinical work so that we can start to learn from each other, we should tell each other when we have come across an interesting article which has implications for treatment.

When asked for a solution, the group first responded by holding on to the problem, as they had just got it out into the open and felt bullied by the consultant's impatience to achieve some concrete results quickly. People will move at the pace at which they can internalise the change. A few exchanges later, someone said that meeting times were filled with day-to-day business which could be dealt with without a lot of detailed consultation. Everyone agreed that there should be meeting time which focused exclusively on computerisation, clinical issues and staff development and training. Rachel developed this and pointed out that these issues could only be dealt with across the whole team and if time could be found for staff development then it could become possible to have more of a sharing and learning culture in the practice.

I asked what would have to change and what would have to go for this to happen. This question caused a lot of disturbance in the group. The energy that was available for change became clearly and suddenly visible and so did the fact that this energy existed in an unharnessed form. Thomas revealed that he felt moved by what was being said and that he would quite like to get involved in bringing it about but he didn't know where the extra time would come from without upsetting the balance of his outside commitments. Rachel pointed out that communicating more efficiently seemed to require a bigger time commitment to make it happen. John and Paula gave several detailed examples of how time could be used in a different way now, how control could be exercised differently and how this would make the time that the group was looking for.

Stephen interjected that all these questions were linked with the starting point for these groups. 'We need to ask where we are going, we need to clarify what caring for patients means to the whole group and for each one of us, and above all what the role of finance is in all of this.' Other group members linked this with the workload and its distribution. One of the unspoken assumptions in the practice was that some people took non-clinical work home and others did not. No one really disagreed that there was a tension between clinical and non-clinical work and that everyone had nominally the same clinical workload but not the same non-clinical burden; everyone felt that this needed to be looked at and adjusted.

When I asked what was stopping the partners looking at the financial and business aspects of the practice together, the group began to focus on John and Wendy as the impersonations of the projected problems and solutions. It was pointed out that the practice manager wanted control and got defensive when it was threatened. For example, she didn't want to participate in these groups because she had had a bad group experience in the past. John's propensity to take over business and financial matters was also quickly highlighted by discussing the recent refurbishment of the building.

When I asked what the rest of the group contributed to the unfair contribution of management and finance work, some of the projections were taken off John and Wendy and the problem was owned by all members of the group. It emerged that the equitable distribution of the work and a proper appreciation of the management task were considered to be dangerous topics containing explosive issues which could threaten the cherished ideals of a practice which was first and foremost dedicated to the patients and not the partners and staff.

Someone suggested that:

> Management is undervalued because we are so dedicated to serving the patients that we are unable to say that we can't cope. Consequently, we are too reticent in buying in a locum to free up time for some of the tasks that we have identified today as important.

Everyone agreed that it would be sensible to set up a back-up system. This was another point in the group process when I could move forward but before I had a chance, the group had shifted again and ensured that we could stay with the problem a bit longer. It is important for facilitators to adjust to this propensity to hold on to the bad object in the group as it is both a defence and a communication. Staying with the problem communicates that not everyone is ready yet to move on. Doing so irrespective of the resistance communicated would imply that the group is not held by the leader and will need to regress if the process is falsely accelerated to ensure sufficient levels of safety. I therefore held back and trusted the group to shift itself to a different place by exploring another problem connected with the underlying theme. The group was also struggling with how to move from an unconscious and mindless reliance upon each other to a more conscious way of relating in a team that is aware of its interdependence and interconnectedness.

To relate more consciously in a team requires a more rational and calculated deployment of the internal resources of each team member in relation to the others. Not surprisingly, the group therefore returned to the theme of money. Again, it was Stephen who shaped the agenda as it was another item he had been sitting on. He burst into the open space within the group with the following analysis: 'The financial agendas need to come out because that is what constitutes the real difference between us. Some of us are keen to keep up income rather than reduce workload.' I asked who he meant when he said that. I suggested that if he felt safe enough he should name names and make the communication as honest as possible. We agreed that this is something we needed to learn during this process. 'I know that John and Anna need to keep the income for personal reasons and therefore want the practice to be financially successful. Rachel and I could bear a slight loss of income.' John interrupted him and pointed out that a reduction in income did not follow from a reduction in the workload. Thomas said emphatically: 'My time is more valuable than my income.'

It is interesting to note that the finance issue was brought into the group and dealt with exclusively by those practice members who attended the private prayer meetings. It was the other subgroup, the non-attenders of the prayer meetings who, feeling excluded, shifted the attention away from finance again by pointing out that there was also a need to educate the patients. Hilda pointed out that the shared lists lead to one doctor being played off against another and how this led to resentment building up between the partners. A recent example of this happening was then discussed and analysed in some detail. From this, it emerged that it is sometimes the doctor who needs the patient and that this dynamic surfaces in some partners wanting to be friends with their patients rather than keep their distance.

I linked this to the difficulty the partner group had being straight enough to discuss difficult topics very openly and honestly without fear of loss of face or reprisals. In turn, this raised the question of what they as a group could begin to take charge of before people started to rush into re-educating their patients.

The group ended with a list of the first steps in taking control in a different way. It was agreed that a locum should be brought in to free one or two partners to design a back-up system and that anyone could buy in locum cover at night without further consultation. It was also agreed that it would be sensible to move to a system of identifying a lead person for each management area and have a second partner act as cover for him or her. Rachel was suggested as the shadow for John on financial matters and John as the cover for Hilda on personnel issues. John and Rachel were then delegated to deal with the problem person in the group of nurses and it was agreed that the link between the partners and the practice manager needed readjusting to include a day-to-day operational management dimension. In the medium term, partners confirmed their commonly held belief that they wanted to look at stress in the practice in greater depth and work out which causes were external and which were internal. Furthermore, they made a commitment to share their perspective on the next five years of the practice with or without an external consultant.

Group 3

Again, I kicked off by asking what was left over from last week and what had happened in the intervening week. The group seemed full of energy, like a good school class with something exciting to tell the teacher. Three decisions had been picked up from the last group and implemented during the week and people felt as if they had put some burden down. They acted upon the decision to get a locum in to provide cover at night, they had temporarily shut their lists until they were clearer where they were going and, most importantly, they had stopped appeasing the 'difficult' member of the nurse team and delegated two partners to confront her. To everyone's surprise, the person concerned had found it a relief to be read the riot act and responded with more output when a boundary was put around her behaviour by someone in authority. This act had broken the prison wall of politeness and opened up a space for the creative use of aggressive energy in the group. It had become permissible for two partners to form a parental couple and temporarily treat a member of the staff team in the child position. Not too much, but enough to encourage further development by reasserting authority through recognition, acceptance and projected expectation for change.

I asked whether there was another problem they could pick up in this session. Everyone said that they had already talked in the week about looking at the workload in the group. From my point of view this was an important shift as it signified that the group was no longer just something to be feared but was now perceived as a resource for help and mutual support. The good and the bad group had been integrated and, therefore, adult relationships and forms of communication were more sustainable. Returning to the workload, the group quickly found common ground: working practices were historical and had not yet linked in with the new building and the current space allocation. It was necessary to review the whole workload and identify the pressure points of the day, the lulls in the day and the availability of staff. It was suggested and agreed that the practice should, in line with neighbouring practices, shut over lunch and use this space to clear the backlog of paperwork and start the essential review and planning work. It was also agreed that the new-found courage to confront thorny questions should be carried over into this process.

I made an interpretation at this point and suggested that the decision to shut for lunch and the confrontation of the underperforming nurse were linked and signified an important learning point. The partners had embraced the task of boundary management by overcoming their fear of rejection when any aggression was displayed. Events had shown that plain speaking acted as a motivator for the struggling nurse and by shutting for lunch, the group was communicating to patients that the resources within the practice were limited and that they had to limit their demands to a manageable level. I pointed out that symbolic acts speak louder than words. What is important is that the group learns to communicate on the different levels available within a network of relationships: words, actions, silence, restraint, partnership and diplomacy.

During this part of the group session I was also wondering what this discussion would have been like if the practice manager had been present and why these sessions had been unconsciously organised by the partners to coincide with her holidays. What was the dynamic process that went on here and how did it relate to power relations in the group? It was noticeable that together with the shift in the group, there was now a sense of taking charge of the practice and staff. Up till now it had always appeared that the staff belonged to the practice manager and the patients, the building and the business to the doctors. This boundary of ownership had opened up in this session; information and responsibility could be held within a role boundary but could also move across the boundary into the group as a whole.

In this session the group was justifiably celebrating having moved on; it had overcome the shame of revealing itself as less than perfect in the eyes of the stranger. I let the group revel in its sense of triumph because it projected a new self-ideal onto the invisible mirror of the group matrix. Only by letting the developing child within triumph in this way can the adult who houses this inner child take in the sense of self-satisfaction and pleasure in being recognised and praised by the parent who leads the group. This narcissistic self-affirmation is a precondition for the readjustment or re-creation of the adult self as we move through the life cycle. This group was in the middle of a transition from one sense of professional identity to another. From my point of view, the group was struggling with letting go of the idealistic view of the GP role that binds the doctor too tightly to patients and medicine. Instead, it was looking for a readjustment in the GP role to accommodate the need for a more middle-aged definition which focused less on perfection and was satisfied with doing a good enough job and balancing work with life.

Because the members were sitting, like Narcissus, at the self-mirroring pond of the group, it fell to me to retain a sense of scepticism and hold on to the knowledge that change does not occur in the form of linear progress but is best envisaged as a continuous process. In that sense, it was only proper to keep the absent practice manager in mind at this moment of triumph within the group but not burden the participants with it at the present. Remembering in this form makes space inside the mind of the facilitator for reattachment problems to occur in the future and this will, in turn, make it easier to face them rather than avoid them in the service of a false but quick solution.

The discussion of the workload in the group led back to other themes that preoccupied the partners at a much deeper level in their unconscious minds. The question of the doctor–patient relationship re-emerged and with it pangs of conscience. These guilt feelings were connected with changing from a patient-led culture to a culture where it was all right for the partners and staff to put their own needs over and above the demands of the objects of their care. The desire to satisfy their own needs in order to manage their personal stress levels better came up against their strong Samaritan desire for self-sacrifice in order to achieve grace in the eyes of the ultimate authority figure – God.

I am enough of a classical Freudian to see this as a projection onto God of a group fantasy of omnipotence and invulnerability. What the group had to separate from, in order to manage the workload more humanly, was not God's inhuman index finger but their inner voices demanding perfection, a permanently satisfied patient group and an unquestioning level of support from the NHS. The group had established a taboo preventing any member of the group owning aggressive and unkind feelings. The need for control, differentiation and belonging, which is part of our social nature, had been sublimated. The tendency of the partners to behave like siblings and engage in rivalry and aggression had been displaced by a competition for the gold medal for self-sacrifice. The group was suffering within an 'unholy' collusive and unconscious alliance of their own propensity for self-sacrifice and the NHS perception of GPs as naughty children who refuse to change as quickly as the parents want.

From the inward-looking theme of the doctor–patient relationship, the group moved onto external relations, which was another sign that growth had occurred within the group and people could dig into their own resources of reaffirmed confidence to face dealing with a demanding outside world. The need to revisit the arguments about fundholding versus non-fundholding was stated and a meeting time was found and agreed. Attention then wandered to the FHSA and whether the practice was making effective use of the resources on offer or whether the group suffered from a fear of touching lest it be corrupted by the contact. There was a discussion about the FHSA putting a limit on the ways in which a practice can save money and increase its resources for staff development and non-clinical activities. The group was pulled back into the victim position for a while and started to feel sorry for itself but, significantly, individuals within the group held onto the shift that had occurred within the group and brought the exchanges back to what people could do to move on. Some people shared their knowledge that money was available for innovative schemes and for the Charter initiative and someone wanted to explore whether the community budget could be tapped so that the practice could employ its own health visitor.

I tried to pull some of this together with a short intervention by asking who should lead innovative projects with the FHSA and liaise with the community trust, apart from John who already seemed to monopolise external relations. For a while the group pulled back from this direct question and redeveloped the context for such a decision. Someone said that the practice needed to develop its own community services and that there was a lot to be gained from integrating health promotion better in the practice. A health visitor could be employed to take over and develop some of the care of the elderly, becoming a more hands-on clinical person and reducing duplication between the doctors and the nursing and community staff. It was then also agreed that the practice wanted to develop a better service in the field of mental health and that it would be politically smart to start preparing the ground by making a bid for a community-based psychiatric nurse. However, people did not agree on this and the enthusiasts accepted a compromise that they should wait and see where the politics of the NHS were going and whether hidden agendas were going to become clear.

I intervened at this stage and pointed out that the group had also adopted a wait-and-see attitude when it came to volunteering a lead person for these changes. Sometimes this was wise but often it was an avoidance of risk taking. Risk taking always involved the potential for getting things wrong and being rejected by other group members. On the other hand, none of us would develop if we did not make mistakes that we could learn from; only by reviewing mistakes within a team context could the partner group itself become more trusting and confident. It was important to dwell on the topics just discussed and trust the process to show us all a solution or compromise with which everyone could live. There was a longish silence after this intervention and then someone said that there were still two other issues to be dealt with but that there wasn't enough time left. One was the rift between the morning and the afternoon staff and the other was the issue of the LOT workshop that was coming up.

Looking at my watch, I invited people to bring the problem of the shift handover back the following week and spend the remainder of this group session on deciding whether the practice wanted to send people on the LOT workshop and if so, whom. Very quickly, it was decided that Stephen should take the lead on this and people insisted that the away-days could only work if the practice manager went with Stephen and they were accompanied by a strong representative sample of the whole PHCT. It was agreed that the decision to go had to be made later as Wendy had to be consulted first. Someone then pointed out that she was uneasy in groups and reluctant to go on training courses. This had been a problem in the past and it would be one now. On this note the group ended. The group itself had remembered the absent member and reintegrated the team in their minds. This illustrates an important aspect of group development and leadership. What I had held in mind for the group was picked up again within the time boundary and linked to what had gone on. In this way, the unconscious mind of the group works to tolerate splits and fragmentation whilst simultaneously working towards homeostatic integration.

Group 4

Group analysts and psychotherapists take endings very seriously and I was conscious of the fact that this was the last partner group and that it was only the second one at which the practice manager would be present. A lot had happened since the first group she had attended and it was going to be difficult for her and the group to reconnect. I had decided to model handing over the responsibility for starting the group to the members. I sat in silence and waited for something to come up. The group did not engage in small talk about Wendy's holiday but gave a very matter-of-fact report stating that the practice was not going to send anyone on the forthcoming LOT workshop. Instead of discussing this in detail, the group returned straight away to the topic of how different partners related to their patients and to their role. It felt like something significant was being withheld.

Thomas had been personally affected by the question of how each doctor related to significant others like patients and staff. He presented the problem in the form of a paradox and asked: 'Will I be more of a carer to my patients if I am less of a friend?'. Others shared their experience. It emerged that Thomas wasn't alone in struggling to define the boundary between appropriate and inappropriate behaviour. A connection was established between the desire to be a perfectionist and being investigated as a result of a complaint. The biggest fear was that control of primary care was being taken over by politicians and shared with patient representatives. This ultimate fear, this unnamed dread, had reinforced the culture among partners of not conferring about clinical practice and helped them avoid difficult topics in partner meetings.

I asked what difficult topics Thomas had in mind. He answered that they had quite different approaches to patients and the amount of time and attention they were given. Some people said that adjustments to the system were never made as a result of a conscious decision-making process. This was most obvious when it came to appointments for patients. The shared lists were making it difficult for doctors to know who their own patients were and invited difficult patients to play one doctor off against another. The group expressed a strong desire to give out consistent messages as a method of supporting each other, directing staff and containing patient demands within the limits of what was feasible.

Connected with this, another argument came out into the open. Some doctors had felt a need to stop giving inappropriate power to some staff. They said a way needed to be found to consult and manage staff differently. I was tempted to ask what this had to do with the practice manager who had been sitting passively throughout the group, only the movement of her foot indicating that this discussion resonated deep in her mind and made her anxious. The group went on to discuss who should filter telephone calls and how experience should be shared more effectively throughout the PHCT. It emerged again, as in the first group, that delegation was difficult because roles and areas of responsibility had not been mapped out. There was a need to get away from asking staff whether they could do one a favour and begin to get used to saying: 'We need you to do this by such and such a date and if you don't deliver we will want to know why'.

At this point I asked about the position of the practice manager in all of this. She responded defensively by saying that she was listening but had nothing to contribute. John was anxious to get into the exchange and said:

> I am not sure whether I should say anything, because I was asked not to before the group started, but I want to put it in because it belongs to this group. Wendy and I had a bit of a ding-dong this week relating to the LOT workshop and all the things we are discussing now. I think we should discuss it here, but I don't think she wants to.

He turned to her with some guilt written on his face and invited her to respond but she said that she didn't want to enter into a dialogue today. She needed time to think about all of this.

The consultant at such moments has a choice between putting the individual or the group first. In this instance, I knew that there was going to be a reconnecting meeting with myself, the practice manager, the PHCT and some partners. I decided to try to confront the practice manager in that session and use the remainder of the end session with the partners to discover what could be resolved for them.

All the major themes that had been explored in the four sessions re-emerged in a telescoped form at the beginning of the last quarter of the group session. People restated the need to keep the momentum going and did not want to let go of strategy, leadership, role clarification, communication and the sharing of clinical practice. I pointed this out and then added that the group had worked hard at getting things that people had been sitting on for a long time out into the open. It was important to end by saying what people had got out of this process, where they had got to and what there was left to be done.

John said that he felt the process had been half completed but when he was questioned he modified this statement, saying that the end of the beginning had been reached. Stephen then said that the group sessions had been as threatening and unsettling as the 1990 Contract itself and that the potential for shake-up in everybody's work had been brought to the surface. The difference from the 1990 Contract was that then the practice had simply reacted to the threat but this time the group was disturbing things for itself and by itself. Rachel revealed that she was anxious about the next six months because the questions that had emerged in the groups could not just be put back into the box. She felt that partners would have carried on regardless without these meetings, until something from the outside had forced them to change again. Hilda said that for her the groups had made the potential for growth and improvement visible. Thomas related how the sessions had been unsettling and painful in a very personal way for him but that he was feeling less downhearted about general practice as a result of them. Angela and Rachel expressed their regret about having to have yet more meetings to cope with change and expressed their reluctance to invest more time to save a little time later. Nevertheless, they took the lead in getting a date set for the next meeting, which would focus on the setting up of a heart failure project.

Just as I was about to end the session, the practice manager spoke and made a plea on behalf of herself and the staff that a top-down shake-up should be avoided. A method of change management ought to be found within the practice that involved the staff. I picked this up and invited her to be the link person for setting up a meeting at which, together with some of the partners, they could feed back the results of the interviews and the consultancy process to the whole PHCT.

Group 5: reconnecting with the whole PHCT

The group that met to close the research-cum-consultancy project was very large and I decided that it was necessary to structure the group process to minimise anxiety and maximise participation. I started off by giving a detailed report from the interview stage, which ended in a short overview of the main problem areas and the strengths of the whole PHCT. The basis of this talk was the report that I had submitted to the partners and the practice manager at the end of the interviewing process. After the introductory talk I invited comments from members of the PHCT and hoped that the partners would fill staff in about their experience in the group sessions. I made a special point of acknowledging how difficult it must have been for the practice manager to be the only staff member participating in the group sessions and that it might help her and the team if she could reveal what it had been like to inhabit the two worlds at the same time.

Some PHCT members were anxious and wanted to talk and consequently the partners and the practice manager did not get a chance to add to the picture that had been sketched out. The main theme picked out by the staff was communication and the connected subthemes of the handover between morning and afternoon shifts. People said that this was also linked with the fraught relationship between the doctors and the receptionists. It was pointed out that there was a whole set of splits that produced malfunctioning communication channels in the team. Perhaps the biggest split was the one between the outsiders (patients and part-time staff) and the insiders (partners and full-timers). This led to the conclusion that staff groups and individual team members thought territorially and not in terms of the whole system. A need was identified to think about being responsible for the whole team's work and not just for the morning shift or the next appointment. No one disagreed and someone pointed out that this was a conflict that they could resolve themselves because it was an attitude and not a resource problem.

These exchanges had been fast and furious and full of energy and seemed to end at a crucial juncture where people had a choice between dropping back into a psychologically comfortable position of helplessness or moving on and finding new solutions. Neither of these reactions emerged; instead the group sank into a long and thoughtful silence. After a while I began to feel that something else had to be given before anyone else in the group could move on and let go of old habits. Acting on this feeling, I said:

> Perhaps it is difficult to move on without knowing what people have been up to in the partner groups; perhaps it is easier to share solutions when one knows that they haven't already been decided on in another, secret place. No one likes losing face and no one likes being excluded. Everyone remembers that the children want to know what the parents are up to. Everyone also knows that the children don't need or want to know the whole story but want to be enough in the picture to know how to act their part in family life.

Both John and Stephen were, as always, prepared to oblige with a group-serving contribution. John was matter of fact but Stephen seemed suddenly unsure as to how much he should reveal about sessions that had been confidential. Consequently, he became less clear than usual and began to be attacked. A nurse struggled to say that she was now beginning to feel that there were hidden agendas. I stepped in and pointed out the predicament that Stephen was in: that he was struggling with split loyalties, like many other staff members. On the one hand he wanted to help the group and tell tales, on the other hand he held back out of loyalty to the partner group. That group had agreed to keep what was said during the sessions confidential. It was important to give those who struggled to say things the benefit of the doubt. Perhaps it would help if other partners and the practice manager shared their experience too and then Stephen wouldn't feel so alone with the secret. I ended by saying that group sessions had translucent boundaries. In my experience 80% of the session remained confidential but 20% tended to leak, irrespective of whether it was a patient group or an experiential learning group. The wisdom in this failure to comply completely with the rules of confidentiality was that the boundaries became permeable; things could be taken in and expelled from the system. Perhaps the staff needed to know some of the negative stuff to feel reassured about the normality of the partner sessions.

All the partners then gave a short and precise account of their experience in the group and summarised what they had gained from it. Most importantly, they clarified that it had become apparent that change was inevitable and that they had decided to lead from the front. By engaging with the group in a reassuring and authoritative way, the partners had acknowledged the most basic fear and need in the group. They also reassured the group that they had decided to involve staff as and when appropriate. This dispelled the fear of being excluded and overrun during the change programme. The feeling of relief was expressed by the practice manager when she said that she had felt better when I had pointed out the strengths of the PHCT and not just the weaknesses. She went on to say that in her opinion, staff had coped with lots of change. What would help the team now to accomplish more was some genuine praise of the staff from the partners. The time was up and the consultant was about to point this out when someone else added: 'And the practice manager, she needs a lot of praise'.

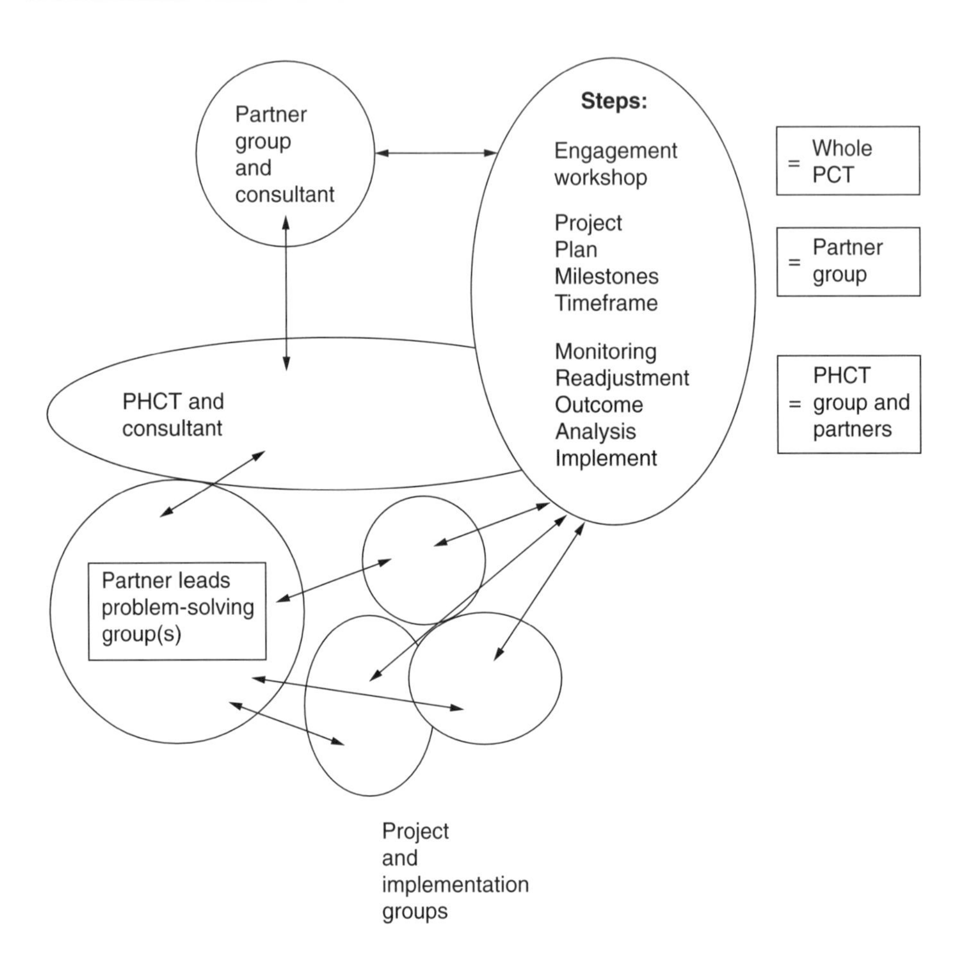

Figure 2.1: A group analytic process consultancy can help to improve the performance of groups/teams and whole systems.

What can we learn from this case study of a partnership about the process of primary care reform?

Overcoming a culture of politeness among GPs

Many GPs could reduce stress and manage their practices more effectively if they abandoned the 'culture of politeness' that paralyses many partnerships. It is vital that partners take the lead in more openly and directly tackling sensitive subjects such as leadership, relative workloads, staff performance, personal aspirations and rewards. A limited investment of time and effort to increase the amount of straight talking among GP partners can produce dramatic benefits for the whole of primary care. Partners and other primary care professionals can shape change and respond to it but for this to happen, partners must find a way of overcoming the split between 'sacred' clinical work and 'profane' management tasks. By integrating both activities in an overall conception of the total workload, partners and their teams can begin to relate in a resentment-free way and unlock enough internal ego strength to face up to taking more collective responsibility.

Slower is faster

The NHS executive and the political reformers need to learn that the capacity of any individual or group to process change is limited. Regression, stagnation and progression are liable to occur simultaneously when PCGs are formed and moved towards trust status. Too many of the change initiatives I have come across in primary care seem to have been conceived in an abstract and idealised universe and smack of a denigration of practical experience and professional judgement. This split between the planners and the practitioners has led to a mutually destructive victim–perpetrator dynamic which can only be overcome by a rethinking of change management and the culture of the whole organisation in which it occurs.

Finding the energy for change at the front line of general practice

The critical issue at the front line of general practice is finding the energy for change. My experience as a consultant suggests that it comes from increased self-awareness and a healthy form of selfishness and aggression. Paradoxically, the impulse for change comes not from dreaming of the future or planning correctly but by paying adequate respect to the existing culture and the past of the organisation. Self-care comes before patient care during a period of major transition, otherwise people end up taking on too much and resenting those who don't. Organisations are living entities and not machines. They are subtle, interconnected systems. Cause and effect are not linear. If you make a change in one place, unintended consequences may arise at some remove, both in distance and time. If you focus on one element in isolation, you are likely to be frustrated.

A better balance between old and new, inside and outside

Organisations have their own personalities and histories. Every organisation is different and has had reasons for developing the way it has. There are no model organisations, no paragon company models from an imagined private sector that public sector organisations should slavishly copy. Organisations like the NHS need to let go of the idea that there is something out there which can be imported and adopted. Change involves going through a painful process of transformation, and adapting the way you work will take longer if managers seek to avoid that pain by looking for magical solutions. Just like individuals, organisations need to find their own reasons to change. Being told to change by a guru, consultant or chief executive is ultimately a futile exercise. It is important to look outwards but only to compare what is different about the inside. Benchmarking helps identify the bits of the operation which are functioning well and should be left alone and which parts are in need of an overhaul. As organisations and systems develop there is a real danger of failing to recognise that making mistakes is a constituent part of life and a precondition for real learning and change.

Self-realisation as an organising principle for reform

People make the difference in organisations. Energy for change is released when people and groups are encouraged to be themselves.

Instead, the reformers in primary care have tended to 'prescribe' how the new GPs ought to behave. Once people in primary care bring their true selves to work, it releases energy to change patterns of relating, thinking, behaving and performing. Most organisations are full of potential for learning and development. The problem is that some of this energy lacks a constructive outlet and therefore assumes negative forms: bitching, cynicism, defensiveness and territorial battles. It is important to view this destructive energy as a potential resource and once some of it is converted to help the organisation rather than hinder it, the potential for true teamwork becomes apparent and begins to form the work group's new self-ideal.

The primary care managers I met during this project lived in a giddy world of activity, seeking to run current operations and trying to improve them at the same time. They rushed from project to project and yet the pattern of thinking and behaviour remained the same. Managers seemed convinced that things only happened when they drove them forward themselves and pushed groups of people into compliance. They were perpetually frustrated by what they saw as the reactive and difficult behaviour of others. In this manic activism they mirrored the psychodynamic forces which were prevalent in the GPs. Yet when I talked to primary care teams it was clear that there was intense energy and commitment dedicated to delivering and improving the service in ways currently known to them. In contrast, the same staff were seething with anger at the way in which others had planned and imposed new ways of handling patient care. They felt ignored, devalued and manipulated but they had not given up on primary care – they longed for it to succeed. The issue was not pushing people and driving change from above but releasing the energy already in the group.

Opening the prison of positive thinking

Primary care is full of sacred cows, some of which need to be slaughtered if survival and re-creation are to be accomplished by GPs in PCGs. I would suggest that it is necessary to challenge the implicit ideology underpinning such buzzwords as health, team, modernisation, accreditation and audit. The emphasis on health at the exclusion of illness is a denial of a large part of the reality of primary care. Unconsciously and consciously, the overemphasis on health in descriptions of primary care is an issue of political correctness.

In the 1980s, as a consequence of pressure group politics, it was assumed that positive thinking was the key to success in improving the conditions for many special interest groups, including the patients sitting in a doctor's consulting room. Health reformers embraced this trend, with its roots in minority politics, and adopted it for mainstream health reform. This pressurising approach helped the reforming zeal that focused exclusively on the creation of health targets, their monitoring and delivery through flat teams. What got lost in this debate is the fact that a lot of general practice has less to do with making people healthy and more with keeping death at bay and reducing pain to a manageable level. Healthcare professionals like to think positively, as it is too unbearable to stay in touch with the inevitability of decline and death. It is hard to live with the awareness that general practice can do a lot for patients but ultimately it manages the process of a patient finding a good enough death.

Primary care professionals need to create a more balanced discussion in which the emphasis on health is matched by a focus on death and chronic decline. Only when that is politically acceptable will we have a more honest and realistic debate about resource allocation and the full range of GPs' competencies. I hope that this will become acceptable and allow GPs and other members of PHCTs to value their own experience in such a way that they can reintegrate their shattered professional self-image.

Moving beyond a model of distrust

The unintended consequence of focusing primarily on health and outcomes in the audit of primary care has been a deepening of the identity crisis of GPs. Outcome research is a bit like natural science-based psychology – it is limited in its understanding to what is demonstrable through a statistical method. This quantitative approach meets us under the guise of quality and excludes from consideration the unprovable aspects of primary care, which are concerned with the relationship between the doctor and the patient. The exclusion of the psychological dimension from the modern view of what counts as quality in primary care makes it more difficult for its professionals to accept and shape any reform programme. The way the changes are framed by the strategists puts GPs in the dock and forces them to justify their actions, motives and results.

This approach to calling professionals to account is experienced by the objects of reform as an act of aggression. This was true in the case of social workers, teachers and policemen and now it applies to GPs. The self-justification required of the profession reduces self-confidence. The auditing system fails to take into account physical decline, mental breakdown and incurability and a large part of the work done by GPs with patients is not recognised. The consequence is that attempts by the Department of Health to improve primary care are experienced as a denial of the true value of a GP service. Instead of helping GPs find a system of performance measurement which actually evaluates what they do well in comparison with hospital consultants, thereby strengthening the morale of the profession, the audit system has reinforced the old prejudice of defining general practice as the non-scientific arm of medicine.

If GPs are to become better change leaders and implement PCGs successfully they need the government to re-establish trust in them as leaders of primary care. An alliance of policymakers and doctors can think jointly about the management of what can and can't be cured or healed. Only in this way can doctors and politicians help each other to break the vicious circle of having a public dialogue which sets targets that cannot be met in the time and space available. In this way they could break the mould of repeatedly disappointing each other.

From a two-person model to a group model of general medicine

The new annual improvement schemes addressing how primary care is organised and delivered means that the private and confidential interaction between doctor and patient has become an object for managerial examination and dissection. What was once sacred and beyond the inquisitive gaze of sceptical observers is now on a par with any other operation within primary care. The consultation has been politicised and, just as the doctor is up for repeated accreditation, the patient–doctor interaction is no longer a matter for private trust but has come under public examination, diagnosis and corrective prescription.

The drive towards audit as a method of pushing primary care reforms through and monitoring their progress feels like regression rather than progress. Before Balint came along in the late 1950s, medicine was based on a relationship model of object and subject, the doctor being the active agent and the patient the passive one. Balint established that the doctor is as much a medicine as the prescribed drug; the relationship between the doctor and the patient can be as curative as anything else in medicine. Now we are regressing from this two-person model of the doctor–patient relationship (subject–subject) back to a model which perceives the patient and the doctor as an object and puts the manager and policymaker in the position of the active human agent.

It is no accident that the special relationship between doctor and patient has lost its aura. There is a group dynamic aspect to this change. The exclusive one-to-one relationship between doctor and patient is, by definition, obsolete when primary care is administered through group practices. When this happens, the patient gains access to a range of doctors and each GP has to share the patients with the other partners in the group practice. The important relationship therefore shifts from being formed between two individuals, reflecting the experience between mother and child, to being established between the patient and a group of 'significant others'. The dynamic of such an attachment process is psychologically very different from the one-to-one situation and this difference needs to be acknowledged and worked with more consciously, ideally in group supervision sessions which would help GPs develop the skills they need to co-operate in PCGs.

The feelings and fears generated by a consultation which used to be contained between two people now need to be held, digested and worked through in a group context. The unconscious dynamic of this interactive process is much more akin to sibling rivalry with its boundary testing, the splitting of the parents and the fear of being abandoned and cheated of quality time with the parent one likes best. The description of the group sessions in one partnership showed that this change has not been sufficiently recognised and requires different methods of patient and boundary management. The establishment of PCGs only intensifies the pressure on GPs to learn group skills and gain some insight into the unconscious processes that influence leadership, followership and group health and pathology.

Being a good enough doctor

It is difficult for GPs to deal with compulsory positive thinking as they started their careers within primary care as second-class citizens. The self-ideal of many GPs is not rooted in a positive identification with their role in primary care but in a negative comparison with consultants and specialists. They feel like the neglected child within their profession and end up in social situations saying of themselves, 'I am only a GP'. Through the political pressures in the primary care system to have a positive mindset GPs repeatedly undervalue their own experience and skills. GPs must learn to define themselves as good enough and stop denigrating their expertise by idealising their specialist colleagues. GPs are specialists in their own right. A reconstructed GP identity will have to integrate organic and psychosomatic illnesses whether the audit system can cope with it or not.

GPs are often at their best when they accompany the sufferer on a journey through pain rather than doing spectacular things to effect a complete cure. Doing is based on the curative forms of hospital medicine, being is rooted in traditional forms of general practice. The difference is not that one is better and more powerful than the other but that these are quite different forms of medical practice. The primary care reform cannot really succeed as long as key players in the system idealise some groups and denigrate others.

Resolving the Oedipus complex in primary care

In my consultancy work with primary care teams, I have also questioned the tendency to be overenthusiastic about the levelling of the differences within a multidisciplinary team. Political activists and management consultants in the NHS have tended to believe that flat teams are better than hierarchical ones. Business school studies, so the argument went, have shown that flat and empowered teams are more creative in high-tech industries with a fast rate of growth and change. As a group analyst, I know from experience that homogeneous groups very easily construct the illusion of mutual support and then get stuck in a position of sameness. In this position, which includes a denial of individual difference, they comfort each other by casting themselves in the role of the victim of an external aggressor or past experience. This is essentially a group with pathological tendencies, waiting for a messiah to transform it.

All groups remain ambivalent towards leadership and authority. On the one hand, teams want the charismatic leader to arrive and resolve all the tensions derived from monitoring levels of unfairness, sameness, exclusion and inclusion. On the other hand, groups tend to develop a harsh collective conscience, which punishes any attempt to bid for the leadership position. In Freudian terms the individual gets stuck in a symbiotic relationship with the group as mother and in this exclusive relationship of care, protection and mutual support, the outside world gets cut off. The group is never allowed to face up to the Oedipal conflict which involves a father-like figure insisting on separating mother and child enough for the developing person to engage with the norms and values of society, beyond the protective cocoon of the mother–child relationship. Any attempt at playing the father in such a group will, metaphorically speaking, produce an attempt by the group to symbolically castrate that person. The result is bad for all concerned because the doctor retains medical and legal responsibility whilst unconsciously delegating power to a less appropriate team member. Subsequently, a culture of resentment and defensiveness is established.

The group that is heterogeneous and works with the tension between sameness and difference is slower to change but reaches more mature forms of being and doing. From a psychoanalytic point of view, the flat team gets stuck in a dependency relationship and avoids the triangulation with the world beyond the family that is characterised not by desire and satisfaction but by demand, performance and appraisal. Applied to primary care, I always took this to imply that I had to work to restore a good balance between difference, structure, hierarchy and communality in a group. Practically, this meant that I took the partners out of a PHCT for long enough to sort out the leadership issues, arrive at a division of labour for the management of the practice and preshape a strategy. When this phase was completed, I would reassemble the whole team to create a framework for getting the work done and accomplishing the desired change. The case study shows that this model works and could be adopted by PCGs to face the issues of leadership, power and responsibility in such a way that politicking is reduced and task performance enhanced.

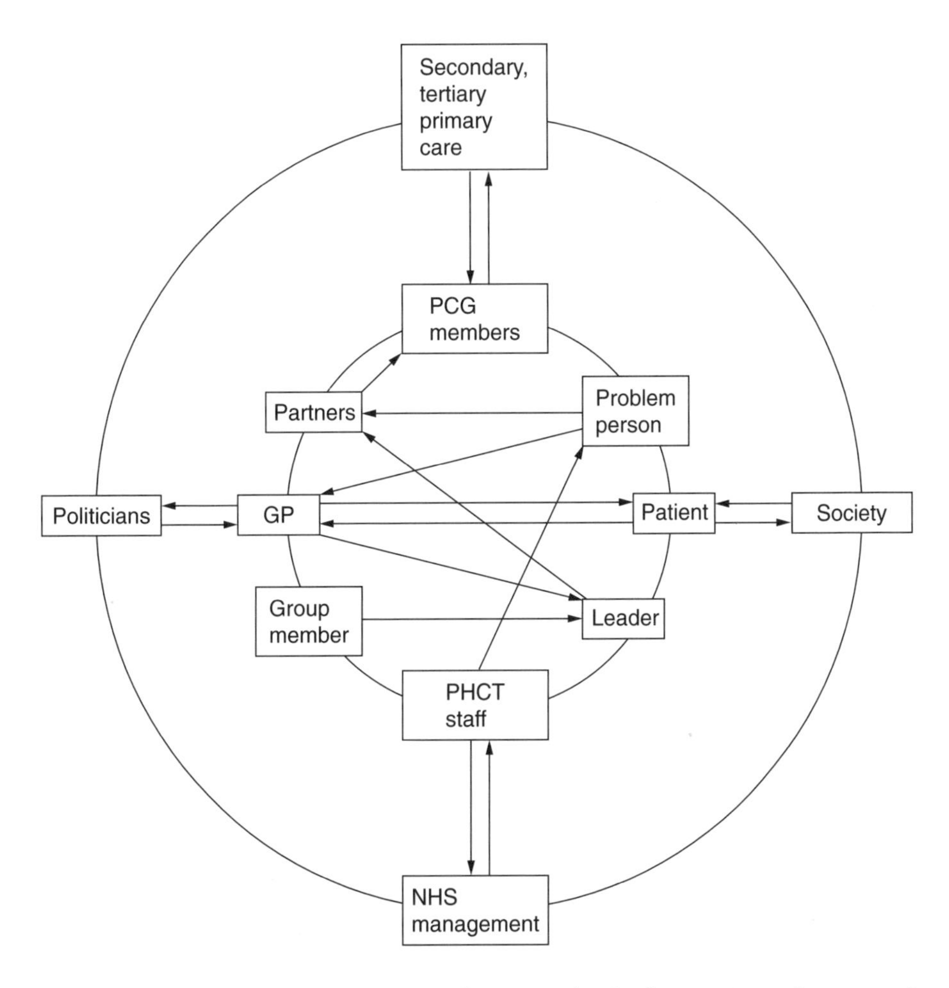

Figure 2.2: PHCT as a group matrix: locating the leader, patient, doctor and problem person in a system of relationships.

CHAPTER THREE

Moving into primary care groups

The inheritance from previous reforms

I feel that doctors have, over the last 15 years, been asked to change too much and too fast and need a space in which to recover their wits and start reshaping their own future. In partial recognition of these dynamics and the zeitgeist, some people in authority have become more willing to offer doctors clinical and psychological supervision. The principle of monitoring the work of GPs through supervision has not been fully embraced by primary care reformers. I want to demonstrate that groups facilitated by skilled experts offer a model of learning and development which would help overcome the repeated fear in primary care that the government is imposing the latest reforms without due concern for the ability of the professionals to translate the ideas into practice.

Looking at primary care groups with one jaundiced and one joyful eye

As a group analyst, I am in the paradoxical situation of welcoming PCGs while fearing for their success. My heart says how wonderful it is to organise primary care professionals into groups and lead them back to their true social selves. My head tells me that it is naive to believe that this can succeed without a lot of process and support work. This split in my professional perception of the latest primary care reform is based on my experience as an organisational consultant trying to help GPs, medical advisors and PHCTs cope with changes since the 1990 Contract. As I work psychodynamically, the split is also a result of transference of unwanted feelings from the doctors' inner world into mine. My inner senses mirror a divided professional self in each GP. Most of them are by nature social beings who look for relatedness and a place in a professional belonging group, a group which can lend them a secure identity and sufficient respect and status. By training and socialisation most GPs behave like single-handers and are deeply suspicious of all forms of relatedness which do not match the doctor–patient model that they feel comfortable with. In short, the relationship between a GP and a PCG will be marked by deep ambivalence.

Those GPs who have posed convincingly as reform friendly, becoming the darlings of the change leaders in the NHS system, carry their 'teaminess' as a compliant, professional mask to protect them from the fear of being overwhelmed by the waves of reform which have swept over primary care. This selection of reform GPs will be tempted to form the messianic vanguard of the primary care leaders. They will help launch PCGs/PCTs and then become potential scapegoats, whose sacrificial slaughter will enable the group to consolidate, settle down and move on to accomplish task performance. I am predicting a normal process of group formation, described in management books as the transition from the forming to the norming stage of a group. These books rarely make reference to the fact that this process, in line with our ancient cultural roots, will involve symbolic forms of sacrifice to mark the beginning and end of a transition – a rite of passage.

Negotiating a transition in a group

If you are a member or a leader of a PCG and need to negotiate a transition from one stage of group development to another:

- do not re-enact the drama of politeness which is typical in many partner groups
- accept conflict as normal from the start and try to own the

natural aggression within you so that you can learn to defend the interests of the PCG and your own practice against false messiahs
- do not feel too guilty when the first wave of leaders don't survive the transition from the start-up to the consolidation phase of the group
- accept the Old Testament truth that sacrifices are normal in order to unite the group and make it work
- negotiate repeated transitions by drawing on enough uncivilised behaviour to allow the group to perform effectively
- remember that being nice to everyone and getting things done do not always go together.

The idealisation of patients and denigration of management

Medical training has made it difficult for GPs to be at ease in groups. A key to making PCGs work will be the willingness of the government and the managers of the PCGs to invest in the development of group skills among GPs and other health professionals. Doctors were socialised into an overdeveloped sense of self-reliance and responsibility that makes team membership and the sharing of power and professional interdependence difficult. The professional training of doctors has left them with a view of primary care that idealises patient care and denigrates management and politics. Globalisation in the world economy could be described as the politicisation of manufacture and trade. The NHS reform is mirroring this larger transformation and has lead to the politicisation of primary care and the consultation in particular. So, before PCGs can succeed old professional ideals and ways of seeing the world have to be given up, separated from and mourned.

From a psychoanalytic point of view, going through a process of bereavement will be the precondition for attachment to a new vision of general practice and co-operative working practices in PCGs. Each PCG member will have to relate beyond the single-hander within and enter a network of relationships that facilitate exchange and interdependence.

Single-handers in primary care groups

The task of mourning, which precedes change, will vary between GP subgroups. Single-handers on joining PCGs/PCTs will be forced to relinquish their island existence and will only be able to separate from the good old days if they don't get too frightened of being swallowed up by those whom they fear as competitors and empire builders. Many single-handers in London come from ex-colonial countries and are first-generation immigrants. The threat to their independence that they think PCGs pose can be seen as a re-enactment of the colonial takeover. The behaviour of the health authority and the reactions of single-handed GPs have a deeper meaning than just the mastering of a primary care reform. The collective guilt of the ex-colonial masters and the need of the ex-subjects to experience acceptance and reparation are unconsciously worked through here. If a health authority is experienced as over-zealous in encouraging single-handers to give up their independence and join in some artificially created primary care version of a commonwealth, this could be experienced in the mind of the single-hander as a form of neo-colonialism. In one London area in which I have done support work, the first reaction of the single-handers to the announcement of the creation of PCGs was to form ethnic and religious caucus groups. The retreat into their safe ethnic belonging group signified a defence against the reformers, who were experienced as missionaries, out to destroy the old and respected culture of the single family doctor with its unique place within an immigrant community in a hostile host culture.

The integration of single-handers will depend on this subgroup having the confidence to start life in PCGs on an equal footing. This will be a question of mental attitude. If the single-handers enter the group expecting to be put into the Cinderella role they will be sidelined and quickly become dependent on being looked after and rescued. They will relate as victims to the movers and shakers in the perpetrator role. In 1998, whilst facilitating a support group for single-handers facing complaints, it became clear to me that this pattern is being adopted by many single-handers in pilot PCGs.

This strategy of going along, having a look, waiting and secretly hoping that PCGs will go away, like other political reforms, is shortsighted. Defending against change by sticking your head in the sand usually leads to being noticed and put on the spot. In short, a strategy of hiding will lead to the loss of the independence in which single-handers have invested their professional self-respect and pride. Those who start leading PCGs will have to avoid resenting such behaviour and treat the need of the single-hander to be in the poor relation role as a symptom of deeper change anxiety which affects everyone in the formation stage of the group. Change leaders in primary care need to find a way of addressing the single-hander's fear that they will be rationalised away. Reconnecting single-handers with the primary care system by making them feel at home in a group could help ensure a consistent and comparable offer of service to them and their patients. It would also help single-handers find a better balance between life and work.

Leaders of PCG meetings must not fall into the trap of highlighting the problems of single-handers as so special that a group solution can never be right. PCGs will work better if their leaders have the courage to put the group before its individual members whilst not blotting out their individuality. If a split between premodern single-handers and postmodern partnerships can be avoided then the PCG as a whole has a greater chance of success. It is important for single-handers to develop the capacity for interdependence in PCGs. This can only work if members of this subgroup of GPs come to view the PCG as a worthwhile love object, which they can care enough about internally to allow it to accept and deal with their need for control and their perfectionist standards. Single-handers will be able to make PCGs work for them if they trust the group sufficiently to separate them from their labour of Sysiphus. The new set-up can be used to gain some freedom from feeling overly responsible and enhance a single-hander's capacity to balance private and professional work. PCGs offer single-handers a space in which they can start being ordinary enough to live with imperfections, to develop an awareness of having some needs and accept help and support from their peers. Single-handers can benefit from a PCG if they let the group solve their problem of isolation, use their membership to feel less insecure and learn to use the advantages attached to group working such as time off, holidays and self-care.

Fundholders in a primary care group

Fundholders will have to relinquish the favoured-child status which was bestowed on them by successive Tory governments because they were willing to embrace the market model. These GPs will, on the surface, appear most able to transfer their experience and learning from establishing cost-centred management into a PCG and ultimately a PCT. This inheritance is a curse and a blessing. Fundholding practices felt entitled to additional resources during the last reform because they took risks and moved with the times. As a group they suffered the anxiety of reconstructing the primary care world with minimal guidance from the government. Not surprisingly, they feel cheated of their gains when they have to join a local PCG which has to start the change process all over again; they might therefore adopt a conservative role and resist the reorganisation of primary care.

Such a situation is ironic and tells us something about the nature of change as a process. What is regarded as desirable behaviour or a positive mindset in one context becomes a resentful stance under new circumstances (Elias, 1978). The change leaders of yesterday become the new conservatives because the situation has altered, not them. It is important that attitudes, roles and forms of behaviour are not just located in the individual displaying these attributes but that phenomena are seen as a gestalt, produced by a group within a particular context. Fundholders will end up in the role of the bereaved in the early phase of PCGs, with the exception of those who volunteer for the role of change messiahs again. The others, who perhaps are tired from the last effort to survive and re-create the world of primary care, need help with letting go before they can attach to the new group and adopt an adjusted role within it.

From the point of view of non-fundholding practices who remained loyal to the old and, in their eyes, true NHS, fundholding practices split the profession and gave in to the false promise of the market and healthcare rationing. This group will initially want to reverse the trauma of being turned into second-class citizens during the last decade. They will therefore regard the advice and experience that the fundholding messiahs contribute to the PCG meetings with suspicion, if they are strong enough to resist the seductions of the charismatic leader. The early PCG leaders, who are ordinary people and not ratcatchers, need to let these difficult and painful discussions surface and not wish them away. The reason for this is that distrust, competition, rivalry and positional fights are an integral part of the group formation process. The split between fundholding and non-fundholding practices will serve as a focal point for these role and status conflicts which accompany any attachment process in groups.

If this split did not exist and serve to highlight difference and communality, it would be another 'binary opposition' like doctors and nurses, carers and managers. Such a split serves as the vehicle for negotiating relative positions within the group. Differentiation acts as a defence because the group is unconsciously feared as a leveller of identity. From an ethnographic point of view, thinking in binary opposites is an integral part of living in a cultural and linguistic universe. From a group analytic perspective we are dealing with the repetition of the original attachment, separation and reattachment trauma which we all suffered when we relinquished our exclusive connection with the mother and had to learn to deal with the father, siblings, relatives and the outside world. We carry these experiences inside the unconscious mind as a kind of psychological blueprint which helps us master new group situations.

All new groups make us very anxious about acceptance, rejection and positioning. Prior to solving these problems in the group by engaging with the others, we regress internally to a childlike state in which we look for ways to make ourselves safe. We meet our inner need for safety by unconsciously turning other group members into figures that resemble those in our family of origin. If other group members don't conform to our wished-for images of them, we defend against the disappointment by finding fault in the leader, in the group itself or with the task. In this regressed state, group members look to the group as a mother figure to make them safe and protect them from the rivalrous intentions of the siblings or authority figures who are intent on taking over and imposing an alien order.

Starting in a PCG/PCT involves living through some of the developmental stages of the young child again. The internalised experience of being a baby is always alive within us. We can only make a PCG work effectively if we allow the baby inside its rights and let it relive the Oedipal conflict. This involves learning to perceive the difference between the needs of the baby (single member of a PCG), the needs of the mother (the body of the PCG group) and the expectations and needs of the father and the siblings (the other players in the PCG and the representatives of authority). These processes are most clearly observed in unstructured therapy groups as there is no thematic focus to the discussion. In such a setting people spend the first few sessions examining the floor, the furniture and the environment surrounding the group. Group members engage in testing the boundaries and the authority of the designated leader. If there isn't an obvious leader figure the group will look for one and elect the person most likely to relieve the anxiety associated with completing the task of the group. The function of the chosen father is to protect the baby from being swallowed by the group as mother.

Group members want to know whether they will be cared for and what will happen when they don't comply with the norms of the group. When people feel reassured at this vulnerable level they will be able to adopt a group identity. Groups spend a long time on the process of constructing an invisible safety net (matrix), which will hold its members and enable them to engage on two levels simultaneously: the needy and greedy child and the giving and productive adult. I have observed these processes in successful private companies, in primary care, at chief executive level in local government and in analytic therapy groups. What all these groups have in common is that they are subject to the normal (non-pathological) dynamics of a group which mirror the developmental stages of the human infant. PCGs will not be spared from living through these stages and mastering all the ups and downs of the process. Developing PCGs need to make time and space for work on the process of attachment, differentiation and relative positioning of its members. This attachment work will have to be repeated every time the group has to accommodate a change in membership. Group leaders can speed up the process of attachment to the group by allowing enough time in the group formation stage for anxieties about safety to be named, acknowledged and demystified. The art is not to rush into doing something but to tolerate the difficulty and to name it in an empathic way.

Fundholders should not be afraid of being envied by those who want to see them humbled. It will help the group if envious attacks on fundholders are read as symptoms of everyone's anxiety about attachment, acceptance and rejection. What the group is looking for from the leader or facilitator is an acknowledgement of difference and a commitment to a process of negotiating sameness and difference in an equitable way. It might help to reassure fundholders that their experience is valued and welcome. Fundholders need to mourn their loss, resist the temptation to be the new conservatives and re-engage with the pain and joy of change. Those who lead PCG meetings need to develop the skill of turning an attack by one subgroup on another into a dialogue about group culture and inclusive ground rules. If this can be accomplished then the culture of the PCG will be grounded in a firm group matrix and can be internalised as a good object by each group member. This will be a more valuable insurance policy than a perfectly drafted policy or strategy document.

Non-fundholders in a primary care group

Non-fundholding GPs joining PCGs will be in danger of displacing their own attachment problems by focusing on the past and the fact that they feel like the less-favoured child of the health authority parents, only one place above single-handers in the pecking order. It might be tempting for this subgroup to indulge in Schadenfreude as they watch their fundholding colleagues lose some of their privileges. Such an attitude would lead to a re-enactment of their displacement. From an analytic point of view this would be very understandable. Many ordinary GPs are exhausted by all the reforms and the increasing demands from patients. In fact, they display mild symptoms of trauma and therefore tend to deal with the pain they have suffered through re-enactment and they are inclined to defend against new harm through dissociation and displacement, not dialogue. Non-fundholding GPs may unconsciously engage in corrective behaviour by showing their envy of fundholding colleagues by overdefending the needs of patients. It will not be effective as a defence against their own need to engage with the latest change in primary care. The formation of PCGs will not be a repetition of history. New structures and roles will emerge as a result of the dynamic processes in the groups and the non-fundholding GPs will have to face their own loss before finding the energy to establish a new position for themselves.

This group of GPs lived in the hope that New Labour would undo the Tory reforms. With the advent of a Labour government and the PCG reform, which extends the Tory reforms rather than reverses them, these practices have to abandon any hope of a return to the good old days of the NHS. The politicians will probably continue to inferfere in primary care and doctors will not be able to return to a simple world where they can just concentrate on patient care and avoid involvement in the polluting activities of health resource management. This group will be the benchmark for making PCGs work. These GPs have held on to the core values of traditional NHS care which was a symbolic act of resistance on behalf of everyone involved in the caring side of the NHS system. Each patient, manager, politician, and healthcare worker carried remnants of an idealised NHS within and was sad about its demise.

The role of the non-fundholding GPs as the embodiment of this constituency has now come to an end. PCGs have to deal with the process of disillusioning this subgroup. If they do not face that task, they will not integrate this group successfully and will therefore flounder as PCGs. Group analysts have discovered that groups change at the rate of their slowest members. This will only be a problem if the change leaders of the PCG insist on setting unrealistic targets and ignore the fact that these groups have, according to government strategy, a decade to develop all their systems. This is the first time during the primary care reforms that a new initiative has started with the reality of psychological time and space in mind. But, two years into the reform, the original trauma in primary care of too much change over too little time is being re-enacted. The government has displaced the problem of funding yet again by speeding up the drive for efficiency and elevating the process of organisational re-engineering to the status of the miracle cure in primary care. It is not.

Non-fundholders have, after so many years of imposed change, still not bought into the enthusiasm about reform within primary care. We need to step back and understand how parts of the NHS and its patients have colluded with the resistance of this group. I think it is remarkable that the commitment to patient care and long-term self-sacrifice is fully intact among these GPs and that their attachment to the internal market is so low despite all the attempts at conversion. The sector has proved very loyal to its professional ideals in the face of waves of management fashions, it has unceasingly continued to care for patients and been appreciated by them and thus demonstrated that there is no straightforward relationship between reformers' intent and actual outcome over time. Non-fundholders have gambled in the change game by basing their trust in the original NHS vision and not in the latest trends in organisational development. In the light of the sheer number of reforms over the last decade (all of which were announced as the answer and none of which provided it) there is perhaps as much wisdom in this stance as there was in the willingness of the fundholders to put their trust in the new forms of public management. The commercial refusniks among GPs did not just act out of romantic idealism. I would guess they were driven to defend their ideals by their own personality structure, the group dynamics in their partner group, their internalised medical training and the projective pressures from patients and health professionals who were fed up with the confusion and chaos caused by the repeated restructuring exercises.

Freud recognised the dual nature of our attachment to social and moral ideals. The ideals we hold serve a constructive and destructive role. They lend us a sense of identity, which enables us to serve a higher cause, but they can also become a mental straitjacket. Non-fundholding GPs remained true to their received ideals of medicine and patient care. The negative side of this was that the ideals acted like an internal prison warder who threatened them with symbolic punishment every time they thought of giving up these ideals or wished to put their own interests before those of the patient.

This overattachment to ideals is a kind of professional deformation among ordinary GPs and could be diagnosed as helper syndrome. The symptoms are that GPs can no longer express their own needs and wishes. Instead, they only recognise the needs of others who are perceived as more deserving. The trouble is that their own needs and wishes do not go away through this conjuring trick; they are merely repressed and driven into the unconscious mind which will then push the dissatisfied wishes of the frustrated and needy person within the GP to the surface. These unconscious wishes can express themselves in the form of indirect demands through spoiling activities. In a PCG context this would be observable when someone overtly tries to prevent others from getting their demands met. The phenomenon surfaces when someone sets up standards for patient care which cannot be met by anybody. These strategies aim to prevent change and function to deny the aggression of the person who wants to be the good Samaritan, judging as uncharitable anyone who puts the doctors' needs as high as those of the patients.

Very often when a person claims the moral high ground in a group it means that they are worried about the shame of being discovered to be one of the offenders. In other words, when a PCG leader feels that someone always defends the interests of patients against the greed of the PCG or its managers, it is a sure sign that this person is indirectly asking to have their own demands and needs met. They have not yet learnt to articulate them for themselves and it is no good expecting them to do so. Non-fundholding GPs are free of trendy management thinking and therefore need to be listened to by the PCG leaders and managers who might be tempted to draw up overly ambitious change implementation schedules to please their health authority.

Those GPs with a history of resistance to primary care reform represent a chance to get back to realistic change targets and avoid the manic and unhelpful actionism typical of all the earlier primary care reforms. The PCG will enhance its chance of success if change leaders can avoid labelling those who object to uncomfortable change as old-fashioned and out of touch with the times. This group of resisters are messengers who give vent to the fears and hesitations of everyone in the group. If this can be accepted, the PCG will start its work at a point which is manageable by the whole group, not just its vanguard. The way the group and its formation process is viewed will make a crucial difference to the early success and failure of a PCG.

Groups do not develop and change in a linear fashion, moving steadily from a primitive starting point to ever greater levels of maturity and efficiency. Groups are akin to the life cycle in that there are clearly recognisable developmental stages which can be negotiated but at the point of transition from one stage to the next there is a lot of disturbance and at such moments regression will always precede or accompany progression.

Advice to GPs in a PCG/PCT

- Relinquish your yearning for the lost world of the NHS free of politics and resource management.
- Avoid displacing your own problems with attachment to a PCG onto other subgroups of GPs by following your desire to denigrate them before proceeding with the real business of building a group.
- Don't get trapped in simply being the champion of the poor and needy patients and be aggressive enough to formulate your own demands and negotiate for them.
- Join other subgroups in using the PCG to reintegrate clinical responsibility and managerial control and help to reassert GP leadership.

Outlook needed to make PCGs work

- A perspective on groups which allows for conscious as well as unconscious processes.
- An assessment of the change process which allows for progression as well as regression and takes heed of the time and space dimension.
- The introduction and financing of supervision and experiential learning groups.
- Management and leadership on the clinical, managerial and group process level should be in the hands of a GP who is not afraid of politics.

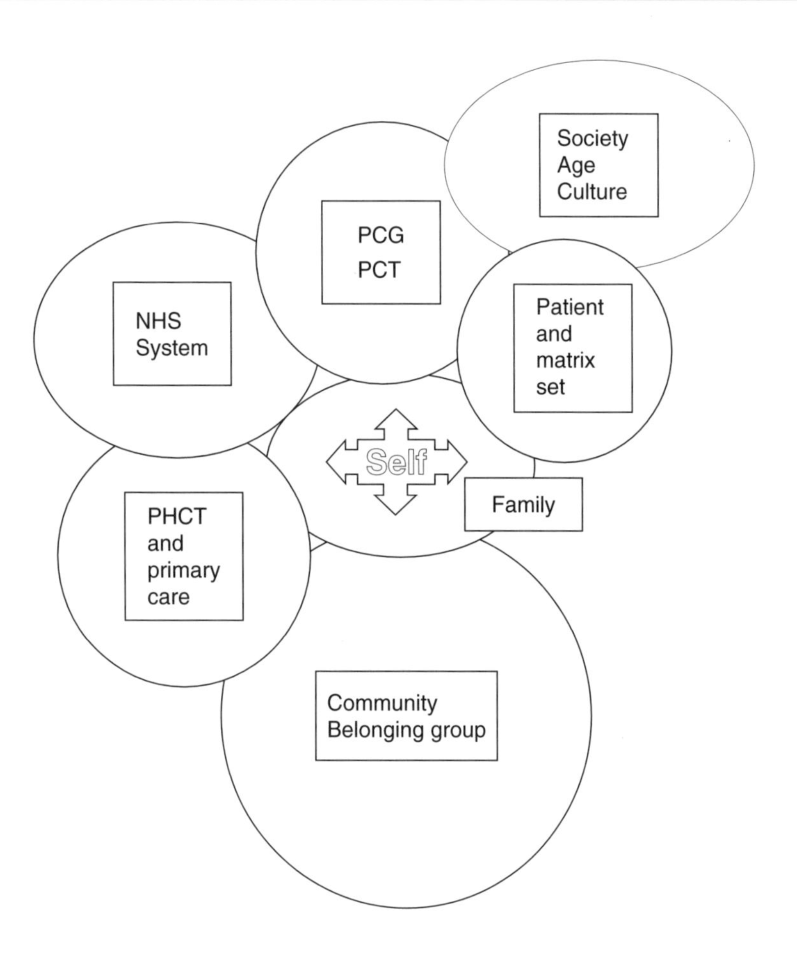

Figure 3.1: The GP in a group matrix and foundation matrix.

CHAPTER FOUR

Moving beyond the fear of groups

The group as mother, the GP as neglected child

The primary care reforms have forced each healthcare professional to find a conscious relationship to change and what it represents externally and internally. I will now look at the psychological impact of the demand for change on the mind of an individual and on a group. Over the last 10 years I have been left in no doubt by primary care professionals that the formidable list of changes they had to cope with has left them feeling overwhelmed, if not traumatised. Intellectually, many GPs experienced the new GP Contract in the early 1990s as an attack on their professional self and emotionally they felt abused. Up to that point the NHS had been experienced as a struggling but nurturing and benign mother.

Since 1990 the NHS mother has, in the unconscious mind of primary care members, been experiencing a symbolic mental breakdown. GPs suddenly felt lumbered with a mother organisation that had turned from being attuned to the needs of its children into a malignant monster. All the GPs I have met in my work over the last 10 years think that the relationship between themselves and the organisation which they adopted as their substitute parent is disturbed. The quality of the relationship between the health authorities, GPs and their teams mirrors the transference feelings I get when I work with borderline patients who have a propensity to split the children in order to relieve their own anxiety. The way single-handers and non-fundholders feel about the equity of the recent changes can be captured in such an image. Change management has to recognise this history and take it into account when building a PCG and introducing its members to further reforms.

The feeling of having to survive

The cumulative effect of enforced change over the past decade has produced a sense of infantile dependency and the fear of external and internal disintegration. Change management has to start at this juncture, especially as the push towards PCTs has revived in GPs the feeling that they are being treated as naughty children, abandoned and rejected. From a psychoanalytic point of view the changing primary care sector can be seen as a helpless and dependent baby wanting to communicate its need to refuse so much reform food from the NHS mother. At the start of the new millennium, there is the same underlying feeling of distress in the whole primary care sector as there was after the introduction of the new Contract. At a deeply unconscious level the primary care infant, as embodied by the struggling and exhausted GP, imagines again that any expression of its own needs and wishes would threaten the survival of this disintegrating parent. As the parent is perceived as too damaged to survive, the child is forced into a defensive position in which it begins to relate only to its internal world and looks for safety within its own omnipotent fantasies. When these feelings are transferred in an undigested and unreflected fashion into a PCG then it will be difficult to establish workable ground rules and realistic targets; the only level at which the work group will operate is survival and defence.

The true and the false selves

If one accepts the good intentions behind the reforms surrounding PCGs and decodes them in terms of human development, then it appears that the intention is to force primary care professionals to be more adult and take on higher level management responsibilities. The underlying assumption of the reforms is that everybody has an infinite capacity to stay in the adult position and become ever more efficient. This ideal GP in a permanently adult position is a wishful projection by the modernisers in government. In reality professional development is much more fraught. The roots of real adult behaviour are to be found in good enough parenting. The baby needs to experience the relationship with the mother as a safe holding environment in which it can express both its good and bad selves. When the growing child can express itself repeatedly in such a way that it feels accepted as a whole person it develops enough self-confidence for life to own its true self in relation to significant others and the external world. Such a person can listen to appeals to behave like a grown-up at work in a more or less steady and predictable way. Alas, only a small proportion of people achieve this level of psychological integration and can maintain it under the pressure of imposed change. The assumptions of the modernisers in primary care are based on the experience of a few 'idealised human beings'. These assumptions are projected onto the whole of primary care and the project of reform is set up to fail because it is planned without the real people.

It is the people who are good enough and not perfect who have to translate primary care reform into better services for the patients. Many of them vacillate between certainty and a sense of insecurity. When the confident self fails to present itself in later life to a colleague, authority figure or the outside world it means that this person struggles to keep the true self integrated and remembers unconsciously how they developed a false self to placate an overdemanding parent. The primary care member who experiences the system as more childish or unrealistic than the child within will react to the demand to act grown up in the false self position. An overdemanding parent unconsciously puts its dependants into the position of the adult and forces the child to be grown up before its own time. I met many GPs who felt like the child who had to hide the need for dependency in order to keep 'mummy' health authority or its local primary care 'daddy' happy. When the distressed baby within only relates with a false and compliant self to an overdemanding parent, then rational and task-oriented ways of relating become difficult.

In later life we still need our organisational parents to be attuned to our needs in order to sustain a sense of self and retain the capacity to use the crisis of change as an opportunity for growth and development. In the context of primary care, when we experience the primary care parent as attacking, we become completely stuck because we fear that the known world will fall apart. We have all been subjected to 'misattunement' in early infancy and in our school or work environments. The early experiences are reawakened as soon as we feel threatened and when authority figures have not made the group safe enough for us to introject and accept, as good models, the new ideas and adjusted working practices. When our false self needs to be presented in order to placate a self-centred parent, who cannot love our true self, we tend to reject any demand to be adult. We withdraw into the position of the helpless victim, whilst trying to please the perpetrating parent with false impressions like cooked statistics, doctored audits, less than honest development portfolios and overambitious PCG development plans.

Our inner working models of attachment and separation

One way of coping with the threat posed by change is to look inward for previous patterns of relating to the new and unknown. In those PCG members who have had bad experiences of development and change, malignant patterns will get reactivated and confirmed. In others who were, from an early age, used to internalising new ideas and habits, the change will act as a stimulus to growth and they will readjust their internal working models of relating to the self, the other and the task in the light of their new experience. Work groups such as a PCG will tend to contain both types and this means that not everyone can change at the same pace.

The way in which change is internalised by an individual or a group, and the response to it, cannot be predicted before the process gets under way. According to Anna Freud, change in the mind can lead to progress and growth in the personality or it can lead to regression and a defensive and rigid stance. The choice made will depend on the unconscious working models of separation and attachment which an individual or group can fall back on (Bowlby, 1981). If false self, borderline or neurotic experiences in childhood dominate the reaction of the majority of group members, then the first impulse to change will be very defensive. For a professional adult the reaction to the invitation to change will also depend on how good or bad the new environmental mother (the group's leader, the responsible manager or the chosen PCG) is at making the PCG secure enough for the individual to resist massive regression and tolerate frustration.

If a person can fall back on good inner and unconscious models of relating, they can stay in touch with a changing reality beyond the self. In such a state of openness they retain the capacity to communicate clearly and speak openly and honestly and they will relate to others in the group in such a way that the group process will be allowed to change them. Ironically, because such people are open to being changed they can also maximise the opportunities for shaping and influencing change agendas which, at first, appear to belong to the others in the group or those outside it.

I know from therapeutic work that we are forced to make several profound transitions as we age. Change teaches us to revise our view of the meaning of life. No change or adjustment in identity is possible without the experience of a crisis. Those people who can accept the difficult truth that our problems are the means by which we reconstruct our mental health in everyday life will be able to grow and develop through the experience of overcoming the difficulties. PCG members with this mindset will find it easier to own new problems, to use new experiences to catch up on developmental deficits from previous life cycle stages by working with change in the present.

The help-rejecting complainer in a group

Those who grew up in families where change and problems threatened the balance of the whole family system will respond very differently to problem solving and change management. According to Robin Skynner (Skynner and Cleese, 1993), such people are developmentally stuck and will respond to any change in altered circumstances in a rigid way, preventing information from reaching their inner system. Such people cling to behaviour that was appropriate at a previous stage of psychological and professional development. Those members who find change difficult will unconsciously experience the PCG as their family of origin and the demand to engage with the process of building up the group as a threat to their inner security. Inside, they will be full of anger and rage but will put these feelings behind an invisible screen to avoid rejection. Even more extraordinarily, they will turn their weakness into a virtue.

Robin Skynner claims that people who deny their difficulties with the changes and problems which altered circumstances throw at them are clinging to a 'dog biscuit' mentality. Unconsciously, such people seek a mental reward and hope for relief from anxiety through attention-seeking behaviour. They could theoretically express their true wishes in a mature and adult way through language but they cling on to the ways of the inner baby instead: they scream, they complain, they moan and they blame. What they are saying is, 'I have to be unhappy or, preferably, the unhappiest in the group to get what I want'. Enough people are to be found in each group to give out emotional dog biscuits to keep the habit going. If such a stuck person in a group were to give up this manipulative way of asking for help, they would have to relinquish an inner claim to a deficit which, in their mind, the parents failed to provide. Being able to say, 'I am all right in this new group, I can be myself with all of you and co-operate with you' would mean that their inner voice can say to the inadequate parents: 'You are free to go'. People who grew up with a deficient degree of trust want to preserve the capacity to say, 'I am unhappy now and it is my parents' fault. Unless they change first, I can't and I won't change now'. This inner model of relating to the outside world will be transferred into the PCG and the defensive stance will sound like this in meetings: 'Unless the NHS changes first, unless the leaders of this group can make the group environment perfect for me first, I can't do anything to make this new reform work'.

Getting stuck group members unstuck

The depressed person needs to be offered opportunities to expose themselves to outside influences and mix with those who are different. It is contact with the unknown that makes us face emotions we normally try to avoid. People who are almost ready to leave their familiar emotional base to engage with unwanted experiences will temporarily get worse. It is at this point that their colleagues in the group and its leaders need to make the environment for change safe enough. It is not clever management techniques that help people cope with change but the feelings that a person's difficulty with the process are accepted by the group and that the struggling person feels safe rather than shamed. What is needed is a balance of support and confrontation. The easy part for a leader in a PCG is to tell its struggling member what to do. It is more difficult to judge when to say something and, perhaps most importantly, when to say nothing. Change will be most effective if the person concerned can accomplish the transition seemingly without help.

Working with the splits in the group

PCG leaders can be measured by how good they are at turning the PCG into a holding and containing environment whilst each member undergoes the mild trauma of extending the boundaries of their mental universe and letting go of existing ways of relating and working. PCG members will feel under pressure to accomplish a paradigm shift in their mind from being reactive in their daily grind of general practice to becoming proactive in their role as a founding member of a PCG. In my consultancy work it has become clear that some GPs and health professionals do indeed see the changes as enhancing their autonomy as primary carers. Others experience the change as an attack on their professional sense of self and as an exercise in political control by outsiders whose medical credentials are not accepted as legitimate and who therefore become scapegoats. The resulting polarisation splits those participating in the formation of PCGs into those who enforce the reform and those who feel pushed into it against their better judgement. Both parties will, if given half a chance by the group facilitators, dramatise a perpetrator–victim relationship.

The paradox is that under normal conditions the group dynamic between perpetrators–victims–bystanders will develop anyway as part of the normal group development process. It happens at the boundary of the forming and storming phase in the group and is a repetition of the Oedipal conflict in the family when the child separates from mother and attaches to father and the outside world.

PCGs will be more likely to survive if some of the underlying splits in the group are confronted. I would expect to find good reformers and bad resisters and defenders of pure medicine and polluters with management tricks. These existing splits in the profession will become coat-hangers for the paranoid-schizoid feelings generated in each group as a perfectly normal response to the problem of transition. The idea that one can build a vision, strategy and business plan for the development of the group and its performance and simply focus on its implication is, in my view, an auditor's fantasy. This helpful, but ultimately too idealistic delusion is unconsciously designed to deny the sheer volume of process work which needs to be done to maintain the group and keep it focused.

Adopting the victim role

The victim position becomes so attractive to those who feel undermined and threatened by change because victims are usually innocent, blameless and, by implication, in need of help and support. The presentation of the self as a victim invokes the maternal instincts in any decent human being and dispenses with the painful and shameful task of having to ask for help and admit to possessing major weaknesses. Psychotherapists and doctors know that their patients' worst fears have a habit of being re-enacted. The same phenomena will surface in PCGs when the going gets tough and sectional interests and personal agendas float to the surface. When the fantasised helper in a leadership role doesn't automatically respond in a protective way to the indirect signals of distress from the person feeling victimised by the primary care reforms, then all the persecutory and paranoid fears of the victim are confirmed. Underneath the presenting problem of victims in the follower role and PCG leaders in the perpetrator role lurks a deeper, and seemingly secret, desire by everyone, irrespective of their management role, to be acknowledged as helpless and dependent.

The ultimate perpetrators are located by managers and non-managers at the level of the NHS gods in Leeds or among politicians in Whitehall. NHS managers often believe that the change agendas in primary care are not open and honest. They think PCGs sound like a nice idea but ultimately they consider that this reform is about cutting costs and replacing health authority jobs. Everyone, it seems, is looking for hidden agendas and complies with sham targets. Everyone ticks boxes to please the system and dreams of the day when they can again get on with the real work: a return to what is old and represents the historical core values of the original professional training. This collusive self-idealisation as the helpless victim is a symptom of the cumulative effect of primary care reforms on those who were the objects of it. Individual GPs and NHS managers have been deeply disturbed and are frightened by what they see as the indecent pace of change. They feel trapped in something superhuman and everyone feels that they have to live out a lie to avoid retribution. I feel that I have been working with abused children trapped in a double bind by depending for their actual and emotional survival on an abusing parent, the loved and hated NHS.

The task and basic assumption groups

Resistance to change is a sign of normality, not deviance, because each adjustment to working habits and relationships within a person or work group amounts to a loss and leads to an attendant mourning process. Bereavements cannot be worked through at the task level alone as they free powerful emotional forces which need to be contained and restructured within a group and in between groups. This process will repeatedly run its course in the new PCG, as it did after the introduction of the new Contract and health promotion banding. Wilfried Bion (1961) wrote in his book *Experiences in Groups* that members of a work team permanently struggle to relate as adults. Group members tend to experience high levels of anxiety during task completion and regress to very primitive ways of acting and feeling when they are faced with difficult tasks and the unknown. He claimed further that any form of thinking and learning from experience becomes problematic when people feel uncertain and undervalued in their sense of self and in their sense of place within a work group. When we face the unknown we hand over the responsibility for managing our ego strength to the group and start to relate to its leader, other group members and the task in an unconscious way. We look for wish fulfilment before we look to task completion. This process operates at all times but becomes especially predominant at times of transition.

In Bion's view all work teams contain two groups in the same space and time continuum.

- **The task group** represents the capacity of group members to relate at a rational level and engage in co-operative work.
- **The basic assumptions group** represents the needs of all group members to satisfy emotional drives generated by anxiety and caused by the demand to complete a task in a new way or incorporate unfamiliar ways of doing things.

Basic assumption positions are taken up by a group in defence against something which is felt to be threatening and overburdening: having to face the devolution of clinical work from doctors to nurses, being deprived of the absolute freedom to prescribe or having to join a PCG. In our minds, change is initially and unconsciously interpreted as something which will lead to the fragmentation of our sense of wholeness, our internal sense of self. This disturbance to the homeostasis in the unconscious mind is also linked to demands to complete a task or meet a target which often extend beyond comfortable and existing patterns of doing something mindlessly and automatically. The core paradox of the change process is that human development depends on stretching our own boundaries and introjecting the new experience as good and ego strengthening. Yet, to survive the insecurity and anxiety engendered by growth and the threat contained in change, we do almost anything to avoid the pain involved in the transformation of the old into the new. It has to be faced that we cannot make a choice between either going forward or staying put. If PCGs are to be successful in implementing change then the groups must avoid either/or scenarios and find solutions to problems on an as-well-as basis. If PCG leaders and managers understand this dynamic, then they can hold someone by the hand whilst nudging them into changes which they would not contemplate on their own.

Basic assumption positions are unconscious and consequently not immediately available for verbalisation and rational dialogue. These defensive stances become visible through the group dynamic and through acting out at the group boundary. Leadership consists of not being frightened by the fact that the real, underlying group dynamic is both unconscious and unknown. Leaders do not have to be masters at analysing the group dynamics but can work at both the task and emotional level if they feel able to study and verbalise how the group dynamic helps or hinders their own performance and effectiveness. The leaders must take responsibility for changing themselves before demanding change from others. Herein lies the key to recognising and identifying interaction patterns in the group which hinder change and task completion. By reflecting defensive forms of behaviour back to the group a facilitator can translate what has been acted out in an unconscious way into a verbal dialogue. The PCG members can then engage in reflection and rational exchange and move to a level on which they can discover their professional self and a focus on the task. Process work and task completion are inseparable and must be dealt with at one and the same time. In the early stages of a PCG its effectiveness will be endangered if touchy-feely work is banned into the container of an away-day or ruled out of court altogether.

Leading the group at the rational and emotional levels

The group leader has the double task of keeping an eye on the performance level and on the relationships within the group. Focusing only on one or the other will hinder rather than help the group in its efforts to complete the task and accept any change. Through regular meetings in which managers focus on practical as well as emotional matters, the group leader can develop a greater capacity for tolerating the unknown and accept projected anxieties within a PCG. This task sounds daunting and seems to require proper training and regular supervision. Essentially, this is true but the burden of taking on this responsibility is made a bit easier for the manager or GP because Bion (1961) identified a limited number of defensive basic assumption positions which group members will adopt in the face of excessive anxiety.

The defensive positions which groups take up against performance and change are:

- dependency on the leader
- fight and flight
- pairing and subgrouping.

These forms of resistance are normal. They are part of our psychic make-up and help us hold on to a sense of 'I' and 'we' when we fear internal fragmentation or group disintegration. In the dependency position, group members might want to block out unpleasant realities or drag their feet and rely too much on the group leader. I experienced this during an organisational consultancy with a practice. In this PHCT the skills-mix project could not be moved forward before the partners had decided what they wanted out of it, even though a nurse manager was in charge of implementing the project. The nurse team became dependent on the nurse manager, who felt the need to rely on the partners. The nurse leader's own line managers were located somewhere else in the system and she wasn't sure whether they would keep her in mind and make her safe when it came to the next restructuring. As a defence she unconsciously denied her competent self and hid it behind her dependency. The knock-on effect of this was that the nurses in her team were rapidly becoming demotivated. The person or subteam stuck in the basic assumption position of dependency finds it very difficult to stay focused on the task and becomes very needy and engages in approval and rejection rituals.

Other team members, during the same consultancy intervention, showed their regression to infantile modes of behaviour in the face of change by engaging in the second basic assumption of fight and flight. This happened when receptionists and the health visitor displaced their anger with the system and the leaders of the practice by blaming and punishing subordinates, picking fights with patients and starting to become disruptive in team meetings. The positive function of this behaviour was that anxiety about their job safety and the threat of losing familiar work routines was temporarily relieved by blaming someone else.

In the defensive position of subgrouping and pairing, primary care professionals cope with the stress of change by forming uniprofessional defence leagues and private pairings. People disengage from public dialogue and communicate about things that really matter to them through gossip channels. They gather informally in caucus meetings, in the practice corridors or over coffee, to plan how to sabotage business meetings. Afterwards they share their disapproval of the decisions that have been made. To avoid guilt feelings and deny their own aggression, people in this frame of mind withdraw to the moral high ground. They pose as the defender of true patient care and start devaluing other group members who try to balance looking after patients with managerial and external relations work. Unconsciously, this behaviour functions to obscure a damaged sense of self-worth and the fear of not being able to cope with any demand which exceeds the core task. If someone forms a self-idealising subgroup that derives its sense of self-worth from devaluing another subgroup then co-operation and interdependence become unattainable goals. Group members stop relating across the imagined barriers within the group and no longer learn from experience. Instead, a paranoid mindset is adopted. When primary care becomes dominated by such a denial of reality the whole group becomes introverted and cut off – the world is divided into good insiders and bad outsiders.

Regression, abdication of responsibility and resistance are observable during any process of instituting new forms of organisation and must be expected. Regression has to be accepted as an entitlement of any PCG member. When the co-ordinators of PCGs implement their reforms with little regard for the needs and wishes of those who are the object of these changes, then those who are meant to form the PCGs might end up feeling dehumanised. They will start to complain in violent and abusive terms about the invasion of their territory. The relationship between uniprofessional groups within a PHCT and key players in the PCG will increasingly be described in terms of the abuser and the abused. Both the change implementers and the recipients of change will begin to present themselves as shell-shocked and traumatised and their interactions will be characterised by high levels of anxiety, distress and distrust. In response to these levels of anxiety and the sense of impending disintegration in the self and the system, many professionals could get stuck in a helpless and angry inner state. They will escape this inner turmoil by fleeing into a re-enactment of the original trauma of the 1990 Contract: the trauma of having too much change imposed in too short a time and by leaders without legitimate authority. In psychological terms this reservoir of uncertainty and disorientation is a breeding ground for authoritarian patterns of behaviour. If charismatic leaders begin to dominate PCGs then the group will dwell in a paranoid-schizoid universe of dependency and seek simple and magical solutions and external enemies.

Charismatic or good enough leaders in primary care

PCGs need to look to a democratic profile in their leaders to avoid the unconscious slide into dependency on the messianic leader. The authoritarian leader rules through force of persuasion, splits the group and promises easy solutions, unconsciously ensuring that the group is preoccupied with compliance. The resentment of the benign dictator is displaced through hatred of external and internal enemies rather than sublimated through the accomplishment of complex tasks and the formation of co-operative partnerships. With a charismatic leader, the group will be involved in empire building to the point of open conflict over patients, territories and resources. The flight from a chaotic and complex reality into a dependency relationship with a charismatic leader represents an attempt to keep a lost Golden Age alive and return to a time of innocence, a time when a doctor was respected as a professional and could concentrate on treating patients. Once this flight into a fantasised alternative to the PCG reality has started, it becomes increasingly difficult to return to the here and now and face it in the adult position. It is only momentarily tolerable to inhabit the messy and frustrating everydayness of general practice.

In this state of mind doctors withdraw into the victim position and split off all that is bad and unwanted in their own mind and project it onto idealised scapegoats and perpetrators outside the group: patients, politicians, colleagues, the health authority. They denigrate some of their patients, using such terms as heart-sink patients or the worried-well, they develop sexualised and abusive language to describe community care cases who they think should be managed by the secondary or tertiary sector. When GPs in this mental state face a difficult patient they experience this patient as a direct threat to their sense of professional self. This increased uncertainty may affect the doctor–patient relationship by making the doctor more susceptible to the unconscious transference material which the patient brings to the consulting room. In turn, the GP will internalise this disturbing material from a patient and seek to dump it on colleagues in the next PCG meeting by becoming the heart-sink patient.

The leadership of PCGs will offer a chance to redefine the roles, the co-operative links and the issue of power between primary care professionals. This reform opens up a space for GPs to retake the power attached to leadership whilst retaining the legal responsibility for the well-being of patients. What is different about this reform is that it offers GPs time in which to digest the change needed to work within the new framework, providing the original promise of several stages spread over a decade is adhered to. It is important that PCGs take the 10 years offered for implementation and resist the temptation to be competitive in order to show up their neighbour or please the imagined NHS parent organisation by rushing into the creation of PCTs.

It is equally important that they don't get trapped in a thesis of new is bad and an antithesis of old is good, but look for a synthesis in the clash between old and new. Hegel (*see* Höffe, 1981) envisaged change as a dialectical process in which thesis and antithesis clashed and, in a rational and progressive outcome, the best of the old and the new were retained and integrated in the synthesis of the present. A similar scenario is imaginable in PCGs if their leaders resist the temptation to perceive themselves as the drivers of change, forcing the passive followers in their PCG to adopt a plan which the leaders, with their powerful allies in the health authority, have predetermined.

My experience of organisational consultancy in the private and public sector has taught me that people in groups don't change according to anybody's plan but by feeding their problems, worries and fears into the group and trusting it to change everyone involved. The group has a more objective view of us than we possess. This holds for leaders, individual followers and subgroups. Making a PCG work and making leadership within it effective involves working on a plan for change but remaining flexible about its implementation. A rigid adherence to the implementation schedule deprives us of the opportunity to learn from the unintended consequences of intended reform. The adoption of a mechanistic approach to change management is a defence against coping with what we fear and find confusing. The search for predictability avoids the risks which we need to take in order to face up to what is really new and uncertain.

Leadership is the key to change in groups as leaders are responsible for regulating the link between the inside and outside world: they are the guardians of the boundary. A good enough PCG leader will resist pressure from the outside to see the activities within the PCG only in terms of achievement and success. The understanding leader will make things safe enough inside the group to focus on learning and adjustment. Ultimately, the leader figure needs to integrate and connect the work of the individual, the group and the whole organisation. Leaders need to confront the group when it becomes too inward looking and move it on, to open the group boundary enough towards the outside to let new influences flow into the system and keep it alive and creative. This will be more easily achieved if the leader realises that most group members will initially hold back from new and risky experiences because they fear the ensuing loss of control, disorientation and uncertainty. Those group members who are reluctant to change need a crisis or problem to trigger a move and at the very moment of moving and wavering, they need empathic and decisive leadership. The leader needs the capacity to use a crisis to push through decisions which are in the larger interest of the group and must avoid becoming a prisoner of a subgroup.

PCGs would do better to perceive their leaders as located in a matrix and as subject to the same group pressures as anyone else. Currently, the view of leadership in the organisational world focuses too much on the individual and not enough on the process of how leaders, followers and bystanders interact in a context which is preshaped by external forces and historical and cultural paradigms. Too much is projected onto the personality and power of the individual in the lead role and the level of expectation of what this isolated person can achieve is literally fantastical.

In my experience two types of leader tend to emerge in PCGs: the old-fashioned leader who always knows better than the group and the new model leader of a group in which others always know best. Healthy PCGs need a figure somewhere in between these two extremes. Such a leader will try and let the group take most of the decisions when things are going well and treat its members as people and not just roles. Decisions are not imposed but the experience of implementation is brought back into meetings and reflected on to strengthen the culture of the group. Such learning experiences enhance the level of competence and performance. This leader is not afraid to monitor levels of anxiety and confront the tendency of the group to withdraw from reality. When the levels of defensive anxiety in the group get too high and undermine the performance of the group, this leader tightens the grip on the group and acts as a good parent who will be understanding of the members' problems but insist on mature behaviour and performance. The skill of this type of leadership lies in getting the balance right between letting go and giving direction. For this method to work, the leader needs to create a culture of mutual trust in which it is safe to make a mistake and admit to weaknesses in front of the whole group without feeling ashamed.

Working on the performance and maintenance level of the group

Michael Balint (1973) claimed that the doctor's vulnerability in the face of the patient's unconscious mind is not a problem but the greatest opportunity for treatment. He argued that the doctor is the most potent medicine and that the best treatment depends on a relationship between the doctor and the patient at both the conscious and unconscious level. Balint developed groups in which doctors could get to know their own unconscious mind and begin to realise that they had no choice but to engage with the work at this level. GPs know how to work at both the organic and psychological level and PCGs offer them a space to transfer these skills into a managerial and organisational context. The success of the group will depend on GPs' willingness to use what they know from their interactions with patients in a group with other doctors and healthcare professionals. If they don't organise PCGs at both the task and maintenance level then they will remain subject to the ebb and flow of unconscious material in the group. They will reproduce the conditions they enjoy and suffer in their practice teams when they work only at the organic and administrative level with their patients and staff.

The psychic material which patients bring into the practice is projected onto receptionists, nurses and doctors and is introjected by them into their internal world. This material weakens the ego strength of a primary care professional and increases their propensity to regress in the face of reality. The consequent anxiety is only reduced by scapegoating. This has a profound effect on the interactions within a group because key figures can no longer maintain professional relationships and withdraw into their own imagined version of reality. The immediate world is no longer a world with clear boundaries and rational agendas but one that is characterised by magical thinking: it is a world where problems are caused by conspiracies and solutions are found by wizards. It tends to be a world of action and reaction, not of thought and reflection. PCGs can choose to counter such phenomena by heeding the lessons of Bion and accepting that they, like all other groups, will display:

- **task-oriented interactions** which are outcome focused
- **maintenance-oriented interactions** which serve to create group cohesion, role differentiation and regulate leadership and 'followership'
- **self-oriented interactions** which meet personal needs for safety and acceptance
- **unconsciously-oriented interactions**, at an indivdual, subgroup and whole group level which defend against the fear of being swallowed by the group, abused by its leader(s) and rejected and scapegoated.

Summary: how groups process change

Two groups exist in a PCG:

1 the performance group
2 the defensive group.

The group operates and interacts on the following levels:

- task level = conscious group, performance level
- basic assumptions level = unconscious group, emotional level.

How resistance becomes visible in a group

Bion (1961) identified the following defensive positions which will undermine task performance and effectiveness in all groups:

- dependency on the leader
- fight and flight
- pairing and subgrouping.

Basic assumption positions are an unconscious defence against the following needs in the group:

- reduce the anxiety engendered by the need for change
- avoid the need to face and complete a task
- deny the inner rage engendered by the feeling that the leaders and the group do not make things safe and secure for PCG member(s)
- overcome the fear of disintegration in the face of all these challenges.

These defensive basic assumption positions are a normal part of any group. These stances tend to dominate the group dynamic and interfere with task performance when the relationships between group members have become stuck and communication is blocked. They also come to the fore when the group is faced with massive change and wants to regress, when group members must let go of comfortable and outdated methods of relating and working and, last but not least, when the group is led by a leader who abdicates responsibility.

What leaders must do for the group as a whole

- Turn the group into a safe enough container.
- Hold the individual within the group.
- Observe the whole group, not just the individual, and guard the boundaries of the PCG from attacks from within and without.
- Always link the task and emotional levels, the external and the internal worlds.

- Be able to wait until the slowest group member can let go of the past and attach to the present.
- Be able to stay in touch with and tolerate the unknown.
- Be able to think in the face of confusion and mess.
- Develop a culture of leadership and followership which is based on consultation, involvement and open and frank talk.

CHAPTER FIVE

Self-care is the key to better patient care: individual mastery of change

Loss, survival, reparation, re-creation

The attempts by individuals to use regression to cope with the fear and loss incurred by change have been studied in greatest depth by the Kleinian school of psychoanalysis based at the Tavistock Clinic in London. Melanie Klein claimed that people who are under severe stress begin to believe that their inner self is fragmenting. When this happens they are driven by their inner need to reduce the anxiety caused by this to split the world into two: a good part and a bad one. Some people take the paranoid route and blame others for making them feel so bad; others take the guilt route and blame themselves for being bad and start seeing everyone else as good in comparison. Neither strategy really works as a method of enhancing a professional's capacity to cope with threatening changes in the outside world. The way to achieve that is to integrate feelings and thoughts which one has learnt to wish away or only allow in others, like aggression, envy, greed and rivalry which turn the person from being good into being naughty.

Many of the primary workers who were concerned with implementing health promotion, fundholding, total purchasing and the

1990 Contract were in this situation. They defended against fear and persecution by being overly compliant and felt stressed out by the reforms. Alternatively, they defined the demand to change from the NHS parent as unreasonable and resorted to what Klein called the paranoid-schizoid mechanism of splitting the primary care world into bad outsiders and good insiders.

Recovering the ability to think and reintegrating lost parts

My work with individual GPs during the reform decade of the 1990s could, almost without exception, be summarised under two themes: first, recovering forbidden thoughts and feelings and learning to perceive them as part of the whole self; second, the reintegration of split-off feelings which were located in the external aggressor like envy, rivalry, lust for power, neediness, helplessness and rage. During a period of great upheaval in the system, in which each one of us is an interdependent part, it is vital for any person to own these negative feelings. Only when they are perceived as an integral part of the self can they be used as a resource to renegotiate a role, reconstruct a professional identity and fulfil the potential within the self in a changing group context that, in turn, functions under altered circumstances.

Melanie Klein felt that adults who face a loss need to move a part of the self into the position of extreme dependency and neediness before they can move on and let go of a person, a relationship, a way of working or an idea. She thought that we never outgrow this mechanism and resort to it throughout our lifetime whenever we need to work through a loss or meet a situation in which traumas from earlier phases of life are revived. In Melanie Klein's view regression serves the positive function of learning to face death. Every demand to change, each regression and every process of letting go of something we love or hold dear amounts to a small death. Each loss and the attendant mourning process builds up sufficient trust and confidence to enable us to accept ourselves as valuable enough to let go and move on. Only when these emotions have been re-lived can we attach ourselves to a new situation or group in a mature and autonomous way, free from inner and compulsive agendas.

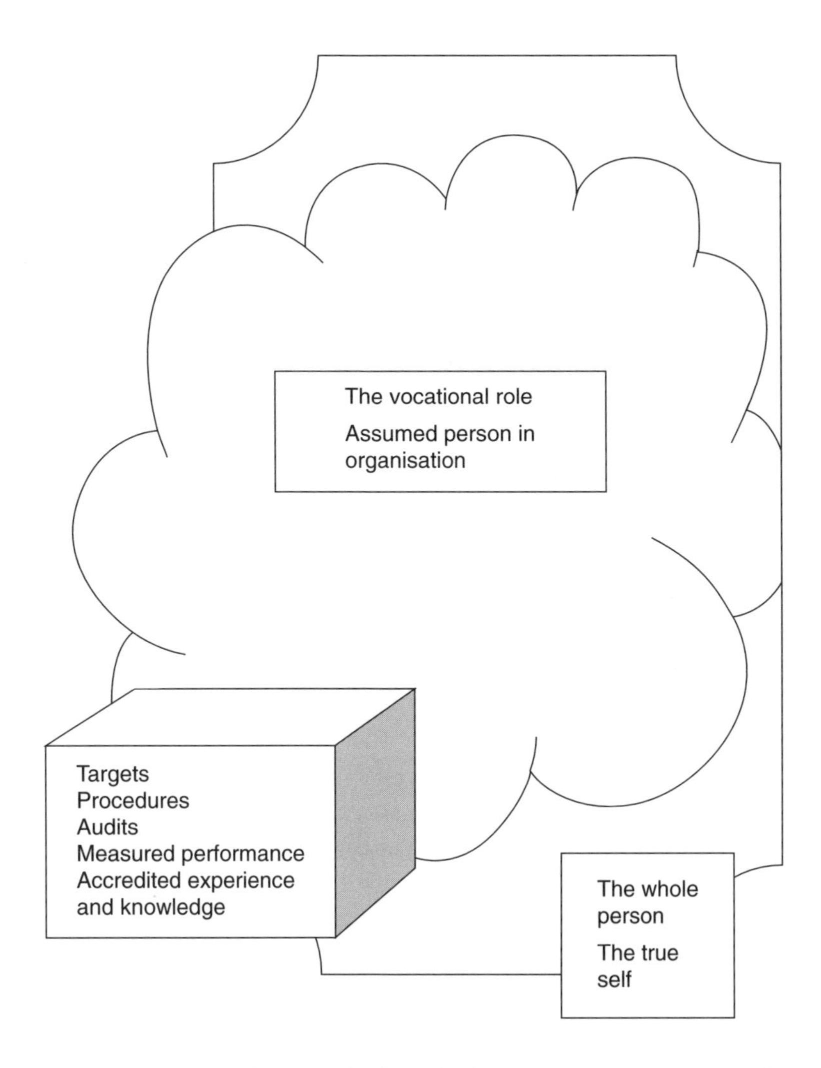

Figure 5.1: Working with the whole person, not just part of it.

A case illustrating this is that of a GP who had emigrated from Africa in the 1960s because he feared that the politics at home were so unstable that he wouldn't be able to take up his rightful place at the top of society. His brother was in the same position: they had both become doctors. The family met to decide their fate. The decision was to send one son to the USA and the other to the UK. From the extended family's point of view this was the logical thing to do. The family deal was a kind of double indemnity insurance designed to keep one base in Africa, made secure by the parents and the daughters, build up an outpost in the country of the ex-colonial masters and a foothold in the USA. My work with the 'East African Chief', as he was affectionately but also fearfully known in the PHCT, started in a transitional period when the previous senior partner had retired. He was now in a position to become *primus inter paris*, provided he had the courage to make the move, ask for the power position and face the potential envy and rejection of his peers in the partner group. Whilst preparing for the decisive meeting during a coaching session, it became obvious that the language he was planning to use was full of provocations which, if used unthinkingly, could bring about what he unconsciously feared: to be rejected, thereby confirming the feeling that he could never achieve a position of status and respect in his adopted country.

When we jointly deconstructed the story, it became obvious that the process of letting go of the role of ordinary partner and attaching to the potential role of lead GP had reawakened the pain associated, in his unconscious mind, with previous losses: the loss of a home country, the failure to become a consultant and the need to settle for general practice. Of most relevance now was the guilt associated with being a conspirator who was responsible for removing the previous, dysfunctional senior partner. The GP became aware that he wasn't just dealing with the succession but needed to repair inner deficits. He could disentangle the different emotional agendas and draw a boundary between his need to do some more private grieving and his wish to take power in a public forum. By acknowledging the previous losses in the one-to-one session, he could re-experience the appropriate feelings of sadness and decontaminate his memories. Only then could he let go of the idea that his whole life was a story of loss, expulsion and rejection. This freed him to recover sufficient aggression to find the form and tone of words which would make his partners accept him as the new leader he deserved to be.

The ability to mourn enables change to happen

In Kleinian terms every change in work habit and any redefinition of our roles within primary care involves a process of mourning. The ability to mourn is the prerequisite for development and growth through what Klein called reparation. By risking involvement in something new like a PCG, we can repair the inner damage caused by previous losses. In a reparative rather than a resentful frame of mind it is possible to create a less rigid and dogmatic belief system or a more flexible way of working. When someone can't discover the capacity for sadness and is unable to separate from a loved object and cherished working habit, they regress and withdraw into the position of the helpless infant. The regression is a way of asking for help by invoking sympathy and protection which may explain why people in some PCGs will develop a preference for the role of greatest sufferer. By adopting that position they are trying to tell the system and PCG leaders that the process of reform needs to slow down as they are not yet ready to enter the change and transition cycle of loss, letting go through mourning and reparation through reattachment.

The person experiencing a loss becomes unable to relate to another person as separate from themselves; they relate to that person as they wish them to be. The world is split into friends and threatening strangers. In this paranoid-schizoid position the person thinks of the self and the other in a relationship as totally good or totally bad. So, the doctor intent on making a bid for the leadership role anticipated the other partners to be hostile and had already imagined that he would be rejected because of his skin colour before asking the group to accept him in the senior partner position. Mature relationships depend on the capacity of at least two social actors to accept that they are both good and bad and that they are separate and interdependent. Klein's ideas about paranoid-schizoid mechanisms allow us to view scapegoats and enemies in a very different light. By refraining from splitting the world into goodies and baddies and by reconnecting the scapegoat within the group, the group is more likely to engage in open and honest exchanges. With the scapegoat in the group rather than outside it, everyone can identify with this role and get in touch with their own internal saboteur and start to own aggressive parts of the self which are valuable when coping with change.

It becomes easier to accept weakness in the other when the self is perceived as being endowed with both strengths and weaknesses. PCG managers and leaders can then learn to avoid labelling and moralising, recognise the interconnectedness of all parts of the system and view symptoms of resistance as an attempt to defend against the pain caused by loss. Scapegoats in a group unconsciously make an attempt to communicate the need for help and the need to have taboos broken. By holding the scapegoat within the PCG and resisting its expulsion into the wilderness, the group leader will establish a process of communication and consultation which helps the whole group and its individual members to hold on to what Klein called the depressive position. In the depressive position group members can relate as adults to each other and are able to let go of their fear of rejection, their sense of persecution and their desire to escape from reality. Beyond a perfectionist stance, it becomes safe to make mistakes, learn from experience and lay the foundations for a group which uses change for development, instead of wishing it away and attacking it as unnatural and alien.

Klein postulated that in the depressive position the infant or the changing adult realises that love and hate are directed towards the same object – the parent, PCG leader, patient, doctor and the NHS system and its managers. Important relationships with significant others are always ambivalent. When PCG members have learnt to tolerate their ambivalence towards the group, its leaders and medicine itself then the paranoid-schizoid position can be relinquished and replaced with remorse and the need for reparation. Guilt about aggressive behaviour drives an ambivalent group member to make reparation for the damage they imagine that their aggressive impulses might have inflicted on others in the group. According to Klein, the transition from the paranoid-schizoid position to the depressive position represents a major transition in the development of every child and has to be relived when the adult has to negotiate any transition. The more mature and healthy person adopts the depressive position in relationships with significant others and the person lacking in confidence gets stuck in the paranoid-schizoid position. In mourning we all resort to the paranoid-schizoid defence but during bereavement those who are comfortable with ambivalence will move back into the depressive position and be able to use the loss they sustained for renewal and reparation.

In a PCG these people have the capacity to become genuine change leaders and can contain the more manic and paranoid reactions to the threat of change. It is important that managers and facilitators think about resistance as a communication within the group and not as something that happens out there, separate from the group and beyond the framework for change. In a support group that I facilitated, a GP posed as a cynic when we talked about medicine but turned into a very serious and upright person when it came to being a decent human being in society. He professed that he had studied medicine to keep his parents quiet and stayed in it because he was hard pressed to find a job which would give him the same financial reward for a comparable input. He had regarded the profession as hopelessly out of touch with reality as long as he had been in it and he put all his real efforts into helping people through voluntary work. As a helper in the community, he felt valued and important; as a GP he felt devalued and reduced to the status of a pen-and-pill pusher. He doubted whether he could, or would, make much real difference to the well-being of most of his patients. Secretly he dreamt of becoming a barrister, to realise what he regarded as his full potential as an intelligent human being.

In the support group of which he was a member, he repeatedly got himself stuck in the role of provoking the rest of the group into a defence of medicine against his cynical and unfeeling attacks on the profession. When I began to protect him by saying that he held this view for everyone in the group as well as himself he began to trust the group process enough to work on the split between the bad world of medicine and the good world of law. I suggested that this split was in him and that medicine might represent the bad mother he had internalised (the carer within) and the law the good father he idealised (the self-ideal within). The father somehow was too holy to be attacked; the mother, on the other hand, was always bad and could not be allowed to have any redeeming features. I said that this made me suspicious because even the most deprived child loves and hates father and mother. So, to understand his split relationship to medicine and law, we first must learn to understand what made him split his parents. Only then could he leave the internal parents alone and make a decision about the future of his career.

The underlying story was relatively simple. The parents had been evangelists and moved around the UK during his childhood so the idea of getting really involved and settling down was internally unfamiliar to this man. The father had died quite young and was not available as an object of hate during adolescence. The unconscious child within this GP had never forgiven the mother for not protecting the young boy from the death of his father. Consequently, he was still furious with her and defined the carer role associated with general practice as worthless – a source of displeasure rather than job satisfaction for him. Hence the desire to escape from it into an imaginary world of law, free of all interference from bureaucrats and politicians. When he began to own the real story underneath his struggle to stay in general practice, the group stopped treating him as the saboteur. They began to value his contribution and scepticism as healthy and gave him sufficient good feedback about his skills as a doctor that he was able to integrate the fragments of his life in a different way. During a follow-up interview one year after the support group had ended, I learnt that this GP had stayed in general practice, taken over the senior partner role and was an active lead figure in the PCG pilot group. He was thinking of becoming an approved coroner.

Rethinking resistance

Change and resistance need to be rethought. It must be recognised that the concern with monitoring and control has led NHS change leaders into a paranoid-schizoid world and they have ended up dividing the objects of their management into those who comply and those who obstruct. The current model of auditing and monitoring clinical work is unconsciously based on a mechanistic engineering model, where the manager looks for a simple linear relationship between the functioning and malfunctioning parts of the system. When managers have found the cause of the problem they start to apply sufficient rational pressure to overcome the irrational resistance. In Kleinian terms, the managers thereby split off those parts of themselves which would spoil the purely rational model of change: the emotions, the omnipotent control fantasies and the need to deny vulnerability and dependency. This produces a primitive and potentially destructive paranoid-schizoid world and fuels the resistance in an attempt to overcome it. This pattern is set to be acted out again during the reaccreditation process and if newly formed PCGs adopt an overenthusiastic prescribing control model through the medium of peer supervision, they will create a policing rather than a learning culture.

If PCGs can accept that change not only affects the conscious mind but also stirs up powerful emotions and unconscious processes, they can make the individual in the group space safe enough for fears, anxieties and imminent losses to surface. When this irrational material is given a place within the group, rather than kept in the corridors between meetings, it becomes possible to go beyond the paranoid-schizoid position and find a mature level of performance over time. It becomes possible for group members to own their unwanted and bad bits and relinquish their medical perfectionism in favour of negotiated compromises which can be turned into achievable action plans. PCG members will then let go of a compulsive and negative response to all change. In an empathic space they will discover sufficient strength within the group to communicate directly and honestly.

The intellectual cul-de-sac of compulsory positive thinking will only prolong the process of building up the PCG. It is vital that regression and resistance are not just interpreted as defensive and that it is recognised that attempts to say 'stop' can have a positive function for the individual and the whole PCG. The capacity for frank exchanges will build up enough trust between PCG members to allow them to look at how their ideas for improvement in clinical and managerial practice could best be incorporated and translated into the existing PCG culture. The individual GP must accept that one cannot alter the legislative framework and become an active citizen within the PCG.

The organisation is in the mind

From a group analytic point of view I would argue that organisations represent mental constructs which are built up and given meaning in relationships. We need to take responsibility for our own mental constructs and learn to accept that every time we meet someone at work we encounter another picture of the same organisation and need to check whether the reality we perceive complies with that of the person we interact with. We project our internal world and its unresolved conflicts onto colleagues with whom we are linked in a group matrix. Through our projected fears in the group, we create the illusion of the NHS or the PCG as an organisation existing 'out there', beyond our personal boundaries, shaping and ruling our lives. We think that we have no real influence over the organisation to which we belong. In reality, every member of the organisation makes up the total system and there are no outsiders and insiders. To make PCGs work we need to accept our interconnectedness and interdependence within the group matrix. The group mirrors our collective personalities, needs and capabilities and the trick will be to create a group that is larger than the sum of its parts and can be related to as an object of value.

Through everyday interactions and the quality of that experience, the organisational world of a PCG will be created. As soon as we start to interpret other people's intentions and translate them for ourselves in a group context, we begin to shape the future and the form of our own belonging group. When we begin to accept and internalise those parts of the change that we can own, we can start to exert some control. With the help of the group leaders, PCG members need to distinguish between what they have to accept and implement and what they can interpret and reinvent. In this way, the feeling of being overwhelmed is brought under control and the need for regression and defensive behaviour is considerably reduced. PCG members must understand that there is a framework for change which must be accepted. When this unpalatable fact is acknowledged the available energy can be concentrated on those changes for which the group is directly responsible and can influence. Imposed frameworks for change are an internal provocation for those PCG members who have not negotiated the Oedipus complex and are in conflict about authority. They will unconsciously interpret any framework shaped by others as an unforgivable interference by an overbearing and absent father. These members will need to be reassured that the PCGs' fathers will not let them down. The PCG leaders must not give in to those who respond to any suggestions by instantly launching an attack on external and absent authority figures. In such a situation the group must listen to the cry for help and ignore the presenting problem.

Management is self-management

Management is first and foremost self-management in relationships and in a group context. When having to complete a task in a changing environment, management of the self is the key to a good performance in a group. It is also fundamental to accepting, shaping and coping with change. Redle (1945) pointed out, in relation to classroom management, that when teachers speak to the individual student they speak to that person through the group. According to Redle, the first step in changing a human being through education has to be taken by the teacher, who must make the whole person available in exchanges with pupils. The authority figure needs to stop insisting on a one-dimensional form of exchange that is kept at a rational level. Half the human being is cut off in this way and sent into a barren exile of non-creativity. The consequence for the whole group is the loss of the ability to be open and playful and original solutions to problems are replaced by safe group-think. Conflicts with their root in the emotional needs of a group member are smothered by a culture of false politeness. When such a group is faced with a reform programme it can only be frightened and respond defensively. Primary care leaders need to own their own emotional world in front of their colleagues in order to create a group culture which accepts change as normal and relinquishes the illusion that life in general practice can be frozen.

This complex process was illustrated by a GP who wanted some help with deciding whether to stay in the practice his father had founded, join another partnership or make a clean break and leave medicine. When I first saw him, I found a surgery which could have been moved into a museum as a perfect example of a pre-war doctor's consulting room. He had not succeeded his dead father yet, he was practising in his room and keeping the ghost alive by not changing anything. His two partners had also practised with the father and colluded with the ghost to stop the son from getting any fancy ideas about modernising the partnership. The fact that this GP had asked for help meant that he was ready to break the mould, take over a leadership role and force a decision either way. The important shift that had already taken place in his mind was that he was now less frightened of the father's ghost than of the rejection by his two partners.

Matters were made more complicated when I discovered in our session that he was frightened of his mother too as he had convinced himself that she would be very angry with him if he dared to transform what his father had built up. In our one-to-one session I described to him how confused I felt when I listened to his story, that he had made me feel that I didn't know whose side I was supposed to be on. This made him think and, after a short silence, he said that he really wanted to find out how to serve his own interests. I assured him that this would be the best thing to do as it would automatically lead to him understanding how best to serve the practice and everyone else involved. From my point of view, he had to separate from being frightened of his mum and trying to please his partners. Instead he needed to define what he wanted, what he didn't want and what he could compromise about. I pointed out to him that his fear of rejection had driven him to try and control the reactions of the others in response to his own wishes by not telling anyone, including himself, what he really wanted.

In the next session he indicated that he did want to stay in the practice and honour his father's memory by modernising the practice and taking over its leadership. We played through the arguments he would use to convince his partners that he wanted to move ahead now and that it was time to change. He quite sensibly decided to avoid threatening his partners with leaving as this would have turned the meeting into a 'tell me that you love me and want me' session. To his surprise, the partners were relieved that he had finally decided to talk frankly and they were happy to give him permission to negotiate with the health authority for new premises and fundholding status.

Overcoming the fear of shame to communicate and co-operate

If an organisational system is defined as a network of relationships, then communication and the use of the self in a relationship becomes the key to making that organisation work. PCGs will need to give up the illusion that they are disconnected islands and accept that they need to communicate across professional barriers and with other groups in order to promote productive collaboration. Dealing with change together leads to 'ego training in action' by breaking down the artificial distinction between the 'I' and the 'we', the 'us' and 'them'. 'Joined-up government' across the primary care sector would build enough trust and confidence in each group to start relating to the wider NHS system and society in an open and non-defensive way.

I was asked by a community mental health team (CMHT) to facilitate a series of large group sessions to which the consultant, his CMHT and key players from the linked practices in the locality were invited. In these group sessions we looked at the common ground between the primary, secondary and tertiary care professionals and identified repeated patterns of strain and misunderstanding. The whole systems approach made it clear that both teams had a shared understanding of what they were meant to do but quite diverging interpretations of how to complete the shared task. The primary care teams accused the mental health workers of a consistent lack of support and the psychiatric team complained bitterly about the level of inappropriate referrals. Behind these two focal conflicts was the fact that the primary, secondary and tertiary care teams all had quite divergent ideas about the meaning of community care and what it was meant to achieve. The group sessions clarified the meaning of the community care reform for the representatives of the three sectors providing psychiatric care and served as a basis for linked and joint actions. Whoever was responsible for implementing the new community care working practices in the locality had done all the right things in terms of informing people but they had not checked for understanding on the ground. Resources had not been set aside to create a reflective container in which the practitioners could meet and check out with each other how the reform was working out in practice. Nor were they given time and money to adjust the implementation plan in the light of their real experience with patients.

Communication is a creative process where social actors give meaning to their exchanges in the space-in-between by making connections, perceiving things in context, linking dissociated parts and attuning to each other's needs and desires. The psychoanalytic terms 'space-in-between' and 'transitional space' encapsulate transitional phenomena at the core of any interaction or task accomplishment in a group setting. It is important to grasp the metaphor that movement occurs not so much in the people themselves but between them in the field of interaction, rejection, acceptance and co-operative endeavour. The words provide a mental map for a PCG because they contain the seeds of a form of human interaction and communication which will strengthen the ego of the individual and the capacity of the group to add up to more than the sum of its parts.

It is helpful to perceive human interactions in a one-to-one relationship or group context as being in transition and preoccupied with 'going on being' (Winnicott, 1965). This offers an alternative to the mechanistic control and planning model of communication in which ideas and actions are driven, pushed, resisted and rejected. The interactive paradigm of communication accepts that human beings are always engaged in change, always on the way to somewhere which they might never reach but which they seek out, when they meet and make contact. The very idea that things can stay the same, that communication is limited to informing people and that goals are reached in the way in which they were set is an illusion based on the assumption that a change message has been internalised in the same form as it was sent.

A change leader who can hold onto these thoughts when faced with people feeling stuck, whilst responding with empathy to the difficulty, will easily build the confidence needed to enable the whole group to face uncertainty and growth over and over again. Change is accepted more easily if we inhabit work groups where the change process starts by learning from each other's experience. Only when this is possible can each individual in a group trust enough to invite others to join the search for improved working methods rather than hide the facts and pretend that there are no problems. In the large groups with the mental health and primary care professionals, it eventually became safe to admit to having difficulties in diagnosing certain mental conditions. GPs were also admitting to succumbing to pressure from the family not to have relatives referred to the psychiatrist in order to avoid communal shame, even though that would have been the right thing to do. It was the culture of safety in the group that enabled the consultant psychiatrist and his key workers to shift their energy from battling with their GPs over wrong referrals to compiling a simple diagnostic guide. Before they could accomplish this shift, they had to let go of their preconceived ideas about how much their GPs should know in an ideal world and, instead, acknowledge how little psychiatry they actually knew. Furthermore, the psychiatric team needed to refrain from making a moral judgement about this lack of knowledge and simply treat it as a frank communication about the real situation.

On this basis ideas for change in the individual GP and in the relationship between the practice and the CMHT could be found which helped both parties to improve their working partnership and through that to improve their joint patient care. The CMHT followed up the distribution of the diagnostic and referral guide with a personalised and confidential experiential learning programme which took the form of discharge reviews with GPs.

Summary: how to manage a major reform mentally and emotionally

Primary care groups need a culture of safety

- PCG leaders need to make themselves available to the group in such a way that the group can let go of its fear of change and face the world with confidence. They need to become 'teddy bears' for holding on to in the face of frightening transitions.
- Change is accepted more easily through learning from each other's experience. Imposed change should be avoided whenever possible.
- Groups become safe and useful when members trust each other. PCG leaders must therefore prioritise the task of building up a group culture which feels containing and holding.
- The process of improving primary care starts through a joint analysis of mistakes and a search for improved working practices rather than by sticking rigidly to an implementation plan and identifying over- and under-performers.
- Just as the economy needs a feel-good factor to function optimally, so a work group and an individual in it need to feel safe and held in order to accept, shape and internalise change.

At the policymaking level, avoid change mania and activism

- At NHS, region and health authority levels, avoid too many new central initiatives and slow down other change whilst

PCGs are being formed and developed. Give the creators of PCGs space and time and listen as much as possible to the experience of practitioners before adjusting your reform plans again.
- Develop and disseminate more research on the impact of PCGs on patients, secondary care, etc. before making a fundamentalist religion out of it.
- Allow for reality to spoil the best laid and most beautifully conceived reform plans. Make this expectation clear at the start and avoid false promises that increase cynicism and discredit the reform in the eyes of practitioners.
- Recognise consultancy interventions, supervision and coaching designed to help PCGs as sophisticated forms of training and make them eligible for professional development awards.

Primary care groups

Shaping change needs to start with the group leader(s). As the leader of a group, start to sort out:

- what you have to live with
- what you can change, shape or develop
- what you have to let go of
- who wants and should take on which roles and why.

A group needs to:

- clarify the priorities and the direction of the PCG
- be clear about what each individual and subgroup in the PCG will offer the whole group and what they want from it
- clarify a process of how the group members, together with the leaders, want to build a genuine team spirit. This would be more than projecting an idealised and ideologically safe version of a work group onto a piece of paper, as is so often the case in the NHS where groups are seen as good because they are groups
- establish a continuing process for straight talking and enter a cycle of setting goals, delegating, monitoring events and

learning from the difference between intent and outcome before readjusting the original goals.

This approach will improve the GPs' working lives whilst at the same time making a space to reflect on the group process and improve the skill level of each group member.

CHAPTER SIX

Beyond Balint: support, learning and development

The Balint model was excellent at a time when the task was to establish general practice as a separate field of medical expertise. At that time general practice needed to meet the patient's emotional as well as physical needs. The Balint model is not out of date but reflects the context and time in which it was conceived. Balint groups were a product of the 'fat' times in primary care when resource allocation to the health service was expanding. In these comparatively 'lean' times GPs are being forced into the role of the gatekeeper of medical resources. It is essential that they are given a thinking space in an experiential learning group which allows them to reinvent their role. A group with an exclusive focus on the doctor–patient relationship would be too narrow to meet this task. The setting and purpose of a support group need to reflect a changed primary task.

In the current context of ongoing reform in primary care, I offer support groups which integrate elements of group analysis, Balint and action learning to restore morale in primary care and help GPs recover from change fatigue and burn-out. The space offered in such an experiential group with no limits on the agenda of discussion leads to a recovery of more structure, differentiation and sanity in the doctors' lives. This in turn allows renewed space for the kind of work on the doctor–patient relationship done in a classic Balint group and frees a support group to give each other practical advice on how to process the effects of reform. People share problems, collect potential solutions and then try these recommendations out. The experience of actual change is brought back into the group and its analysis can start a learning organisation in the mind that can be transferred from a support group into the culture of a forming PCG or PCT.

My thinking about groups and their use as an effective tool for teaching, learning and problem solving is rooted in the work of SH Foulkes, the founder of group analysis, and David Casey, who is a pioneer of action learning groups. Group analysts perceive human beings as social beings on both a conscious and unconscious level. In Foulkes' view work problems and 'dis-ease' are not located in a single individual but originate between people in a relationship or a network of relationships which he called a 'matrix'. From this perspective malfunctions in a group or underperformance in an individual would be reframed as an incompatibility between the interests of the individual and the group – the 'I' and the 'we'. In any group each member transfers inappropriate patterns of interaction and communication into the work group and makes inappropriate emotional demands on it. The group experiences the individual as incapable of fitting in or unable to give and receive advice. The resulting mutual frustrations build up into a regular set of symptoms. Awareness of this inability to relate properly is repressed. The pattern gets set because the individual becomes a 'nodal point' in the network of relationships and takes on other people's projected malfunction. The symptom-bearing person begins to embody something unwanted for everyone in the group. The other group members collude with the behaviour because they would rather see their own symptoms located in a scapegoat than in themselves. The same pattern of 'malignant mirroring' goes on between subgroups within the primary care sector (Zinkin, 1983).

Recurring problems in a work group can be seen as 'neurotic symptoms' which symbolise what cannot yet be brought into a dialogue between mature and problem-solving adults. This behaviour is accentuated under the pressure of imposed change because that process generates feelings of persecution and resistance on top of the normal difficulty of interacting in the adult mode within a group. Communication in such a set-up will take the form of 'acting out' instead of talking.

Group analysis involves the translation of the energy invested in the symptom or the problem into a shared communication during a group process facilitated by an analytically trained group facilitator.

The belief is that if the group 'conductor' (Foulkes' image for a leader) leaves the group to do the sharing and working through of the problem, the best solution will be found. The group analytic process fosters new insights into destructive behaviour by allowing the group to confront and overcome its fear of the unknown. To this end, it is very important that the group does not follow a preset programme in accordance with a set of testable hypotheses; nor would it be acceptable to state what a doctor can and can't bring into the group. In this sense, a group analytic model goes beyond Balint in that it assumes that forbidding doctors to talk in depth about themselves and only focus on the patient and the GPs' reaction to the patient will produce a false self-dynamic.

Group analysts believe that the group itself helps its members collectively to redefine the group norms from which they individually deviate. Outside pressures and idealised models of working get in the way because they usually serve to unite falsely group members around the defence of denial and undermine genuine work for real change. Enforced change has engulfed primary care over the last 15 years to such an extent that the basic trust between doctor and patient, health authority and primary care team has been damaged and needs to be rebuilt. It is the GPs in PCGs who need to become the focus of support work. The future lies in turning Balint on his head and enabling doctors to learn that self-care is the most direct route to better patient care. I believe that each group session lives through the drama of birth, attachment, loss, separation, transition and ending. If the PCG group can follow the developmental cycle of life itself during each of its meetings, then there is an increased likelihood of group members reaching the adult position, in which they can face, tolerate and internalise change and stay focused on the task.

Developing a process model of training and development

David Casey (1993), in his book *Managing Learning in Organisations*, looks at how organisations and teams develop responsibility within their employees by devolving important decisions. The modern manager has to take responsibility for the technical performance and co-operation of staff. The need for self-examination and self-improvement became the starting point for Casey's management training and organisational development programmes. He pointed out that training and consultancy interventions used to reflect the ideal type executive and therefore concentrated on getting things done, not being complicated and ensuring predictable growth, improvement and change. Everything had to be measurable and controllable; the ultimate aim was to attain change but avoid disturbance in the organisation.

Changes in the market place, politics and culture have meant that this idea of defining disturbances as abnormal, a blip in the smooth running of the organisation machine, turns out to be more of a fantasy than a reality. Casey argues that a paradigm shift is needed from a mechanical engineering model to a process model of training and development. The manager's task therefore is to help to make the reality of continuous self-examination acceptable and help to create self-managing teams and reflective training forums.

It follows from this that training for PCGs should address the following questions.

- How PCG leaders and members learn.
- How the PCG members can translate experience into improved performance.
- How entire organisations start to share and generate knowledge.
- How PCGs can link in with the whole primary care system to import and export experience and learning.
- How audit and evidence-based medicine can become tools for developing a learning organisation.
- How primary care can get away from a culture of control, intimidation and bribery.

The word 'learn' can easily be substituted for the word 'change'; learning amounts to changing and change without learning is not possible. For Casey (1993), the preconditions for a mature self-managing group with a manager who can delegate are leadership, self-knowledge and the acquisition of group skills. Mature work groups operate on two levels: the rational and the emotional. Unless the uncontrollable and unmeasurable emotional side of a

PCG is accepted and brought into the dialogue, the future cannot be faced and needs to be blocked out. Groups fear change and malfunction as 'the essence of the daily running of a complex social system is certainty; the essence of steering it towards the future is uncertainty' (Casey, 1993). Action learning groups were set up so that managers could go beyond the task of formulating strategy and implementing the business plan. Casey wanted them to include in their brief the task of mutual support, learning from experience and engaging in informal exchange to build up trust and self-knowledge. All this applies to doctors in the changed context of primary care and will provide the basis on which PCGs can be made to work or will begin to fail. By becoming more vulnerable in an experiential learning or supervision group, PCG members will gain rather than lose credibility with their peers and shift relationships within the group and between practices in the area from territorial differentiation towards co-operation and networking.

The gain which Casey predicted for managers (and each GP is a manager) taking the risk of participating in case supervision groups was the ability to face the future and embrace change as a chance to learn and survive as an ongoing process. The combined thinking of Foulkes and Casey explains why I adopt experiential learning groups as the preferred method of discovering and transmitting new knowledge and skills to struggling GPs.

From a reactive to a proactive culture through supervision

These ideas go to the heart of some of the teaching and learning principles which the London Implementation Zone Educational Initiative (LIZEI) tried to encapsulate. The scheme provided the opportunity to address the problems of recruitment, retention and refreshment of inner London GPs. The Academic Department at St George's Hospital developed a group educational project for doctors in mid-career. The aims of the project were to set up an educational group that would address both perceived and real educational needs, develop teaching skills and provide support. In the third year the project became a launch pad for the first PCG pilots. I facilitated a weekly, 90-minute group session where issues and problems were shared and understood at the task and emotional levels. The group sessions were different from the Balint model as the focus shifted away from simply providing a better service to patients to helping the GPs survive the deep structural changes in the NHS and consolidate their careers. I thought that a problem-led approach to group work, integrating group analysis and action learning, would be more helpful to GPs than a purely psychoanalytic approach which limits itself to transference and countertransference issues. The underlying philosophy I adopted was that self-care is the route to better patient care in an environment of rationed resources. PCGs need to adopt the principles of a learning company and base changes in general practice on a review of their own experience and consultation with other professionals in the system.

Providing a modified model of clinical supervision is the secret ingredient for ensuring that PCGs can be made to work. The previous reforms of the early 1990s challenged doctors to integrate management and medicine. PCGs and PCTs are expected to go further still and see their work in medical, political, legal and managerial terms. The St George's-based (Bolingbroke Group) LIZEI project set out to achieve a paradigm shift in GPs from a reactive to a proactive stance, from simply offering care to managing the system of care. The project also aimed to remotivate GPs to stay in primary care, encourage them to create their own professional development programme and build up local support networks to alleviate the pressure of organisational change and political and social isolation.

GPs were given time out and locum cover for the project. In the light of the expenditure involved it was decided to have a pilot project which would be reviewed after six weeks, before going ahead with a full complement of group members for the rest of the year. In the countertransference this set-up made me aware of what it was like to feel under threat from clinical audit and evidence-based medicine. Although the group had to prove itself, the pressures to cope with the primary care reforms had built up so much that there was no resistance to talking and sharing. By taking the risk of giving and taking in the group, its members ensured that they would have a transitional space for change, mutual support and co-operative problem solving for the rest of the year.

Self-doubt and neediness

The first group session was preoccupied with leadership, authority and the culture of their respective practices. People dwelled on being frightened of the group and envied by their colleagues for having a session solely reserved for their own needs and problems. It became apparent that doctors don't perceive themselves as having power or needs; they gain control by serving others. People said that they were only in the group because they wanted to get in touch with their own need for development and hoped to prevent further burn-out. Fear of the group surfaced during a discussion of how people felt overwhelmed or buried under the sheer weight of paperwork and the patients' greed for care. The question repeatedly posed was: 'Will I be able to show my greed here without getting rejected?'. This was important as a self-directed learning programme depends on people being in touch with their need to relate, their capacity to be empathic and their wish to be selfish and self-centred. At an unconscious level it felt as if the group was preoccupied with asking whether they, as doctors, could ever be good enough, whether their feeling of being misunderstood and attacked by their political masters wasn't partly justified because they felt so inadequate inside.

The addiction to the doctor–patient relationship

The second group was preoccupied with the need for structure and a defence against the unpredictability of demand within general practice. The pattern of interaction and communication was very much shaped by the internalised model of the doctor–patient relationship. As soon as someone volunteered to speak, they were diagnosed, treated and ticked off by the group acting as a merged and collective group GP. Anything to stay out of the sick role. It was difficult to stay in touch with anybody's feelings and it was virtually impossible to lead the group. There was uncertainty about having both the lecturers and students in the same group, a split that was mirrored in the group by those presenting as having problems and those who had sorted it all out. The split into those needing help and those offering it could not be maintained, as the underlying topic of fearing patient complaints and practising defensive medicine exposed the current vulnerability and helplessness of all the doctors.

Support groups are as unpredictable as general practice

The third group began to acknowledge the end of the beginning. People asked what the group was for and what was being achieved. The group split into subgroups. Some group members thought that a supervision group could be a waste of taxpayers' money and others thought that giving doctors a treat was long overdue. The idea was put forward that the unpredictability of the group was like primary care and highlighted the real skills and adaptability of GPs. A group member revealed that his absence from the practice had led to resentment and envy and said that the group was valuable because he had discovered how difficult it is for him to shape his own agenda. This led to a discussion of how important it is to appreciate what one has and how much one is worth. The importance of outcome research was then explored and people found that their ability to predict and achieve certain outcomes in medicine was very limited. 'The question for this group', someone said, 'is whether we can learn to stay with process issues and not avoid uncomfortable feelings and thoughts by focusing on outcomes.'

Selfishness and loyalty

Just before the fourth session one of the teachers announced that he was leaving this project because he had been offered the management of another new initiative in the medical school. The group then became preoccupied with the themes of commitment, selfishness, loyalty and their reputation as doctors. Members of the group linked these themes to their relative lack of power and they explored how they felt at the mercy of the politicians, managers and, increasingly, their greedy patients. The doctor as a helpless victim, full of rage inside but impotent when it comes to resistance and defence, emerged as one position around which people rallied. The counter-argument was represented by one person playing the role of the detached cynic who had relinquished the idea of a vocation and perceived medicine as a mere money-spinner to finance his leisure pursuits. Unconsciously, all this was connected to the member of the group leaving without a proper process of separation. By doing this, he raised memories of imposed change, the unpredictability of general medicine and the experience of being left behind or feeling excluded and abandoned. The group coped with these negative feelings by looking for fault in themselves and several members ended up feeling threatened.

The split into those who move on and possess insider knowledge and those who are left behind by change was mirrored in a connected topic of dividing the workload into real work and shit work, one being medical, the other being administrative and financial. The discussion also mirrored the split into fundholders and non-fundholders that had become a moral watershed within the profession. This division of sacred and profane spheres in primary care was overcome when someone reframed the problem by suggesting that it might help if people stopped assuming that every doctor only wants to be a medic and found out who had the energy and interest for managerial tasks. It turned out that he was interested in non-medical aspects of the practice and would be prepared to take on more of these responsibilities if the activity was given time and value. The practical outcome of these exchanges was that he took these thoughts to a partner meeting and began to reshape the roles within the team. After the supervision group ended he set about negotiating new premises with the health authority, took over the senior partner role and became a key player in setting up the first PCG in the area.

In this session people also explored the difficulties associated with having clear boundaries and roles in general practice. They agreed that boundaries made the difference when it came to time and stress management but it emerged that no one in the group was taking as many sessions out of the practice as they were offered within the framework of the project. There was a common assumption that there had to be rules, guidelines and procedures to regulate relationships in primary care but that effective work performance and the management of team morale depended on bending the rules and being overcommitted. The majority of the doctors had decided to cope with the envy of being out of the practice and receiving support by offering an extra session to their partners. Someone stood out against that and said: 'I don't do that and maybe that is why I become the scapegoat in partner meetings and why you find it difficult to hear what I am saying'. An important mechanism underlying the group dynamics of a work team had been understood, that of rivalry, envy and scapegoating.

Overcoming a sense of isolation and helplessness

The fifth group session began by sharing a sense of isolation. This topic had previously been associated with the single-handers but in this session it became clear that one can be very lonely in a group or in a pair. The group explored the difficulties associated with joining and staying in a partnership. There was a recognition of the need to accept full responsibility for one's own interests and learn to look after them assertively rather than indirectly by using partners or patients.

Body and mind in general practice

The sixth and final session of the pilot project focused on finding better ways of managing heart-sink patients and opened up the whole issue of the link between the body and the mind in diagnosis, treatment and the definition of therapeutic outcomes. In the phrase of one group member, the focal question of this group was: 'How do I de-medicalise the problem when the person has come to me for medical treatment in order to avoid the real distress?' After examining a number of case histories the group agreed that the doctor can't help in most cases but has an important role acting as a referring agent, container and listening prop. This exposed the contradiction between practice reality and the ideals of organic medicine. It was acknowledged that each GP had to learn that being there, listening, confronting a patient and handing back the responsibility to the patient was a valuable thing to do and counted as a form of treatment, albeit one with limited therapeutic outcomes.

Development, learning and maturation

A maturation process took place in these six group sessions and I could see a reduction in the stress levels of some of these doctors. From a psychoanalytic point of view, the carer must learn to look after the self first in order to offer appropriate levels of care to the patient. In the limited time available this group had internalised these values and started to act on them in their primary care practice. Practice and primary care group development must not just be viewed in terms of improving systems, staff–patient ratios, clinical guidance and bricks and mortar. The group sessions showed that there is a deep need for GPs to meet for the purpose of support. Doctors could develop a learning network that encourages them to share their problems and use their own experience as a resource. Finding solutions during a process of reviewing one's own performance and experience encourages the development of a learning organisation.

The supervision sessions demonstrated that doctors had become very isolated and were still the object of powerful projections by patients, staff and the community. In order to better deal with these pressures and retain a sense of realism and self, it became clear to me that doctors would benefit from non-managerial supervision. It emerged during the open group analytic sessions that the doctors' instinctual reaction to a problem is to view it and treat it in the framework of an internalised doctor–patient relationship. It would seem appropriate to integrate the lessons from Balint groups into continued professional development programmes for GPs.

These sessions also revealed that the Balint focus on the doctor as the medicine and the one-to-one relationship as the treatment mechanism was appropriate in times when the doctor felt respected. After a turbulent period of imposed health reforms, the context had altered to such a degree that it was time to go beyond the boundary of the Balint universe. Focusing on the unconscious interaction between patient and doctor and the effect this transference dynamic has on treatment is at present not addressing the real pressure and stress points for doctors in their everyday life. The containing relationship of the doctor with the single patient had its blanket of protective confidentiality lifted and was now under the gaze of the auditor. In short, the most sacred space in primary care had become an object for public and political examination.

In this context, both the doctor and the patient need to be contained and supported in a group setting. The skills needed for holding a patient and containing a treatment programme within a group boundary have not yet developed sufficiently in primary care, even though everyone thinks they can form and facilitate groups. Regular group supervision would open up a space in which PCG members could do enough process work to ensure that their group engages in continuous improvement which provides best value to their patients. Above all, it would enable GPs to develop their group skills which they now need to manage their patients, staff, each other and the outside world.

Membership in a supervision group and learning outcomes

Each of the three Bolingbroke project groups developed a distinct group culture and unconsciously chose their collective trauma to work on. Similar phenomena will be observable in PCGs as their membership will vary from area to area by career history, gender, age and ethnicity. Year 1 of this project was a heterogeneous group in terms of age, gender and type of practice.

Year 1: coping in the keep-death-at-bay service of general practice

The first Bolingbroke year group was united by the fact that they had survived the pilot phase described above and were all old enough to have practised in the days before the 1990 Contract so they all had a great deal of 'mourning work' to do. The loss of the good old days and the transition to the bad new days dominated their thoughts. The demands on these doctors were perceived as so varied and heavy that their own development needs got buried under a wish-list designed to satisfy patients or the expectations of the health authority. Pleasing the system had a defensive function and was a symptom of insecurity and fear. The reaction to the fear varied: some of the GPs were hiding from the changes, others were overanxious to please the change leaders, a third category seemed confused about the expectations put on them. The overall effect of the reforms on these practitioners had been severe role strain. They needed to redefine the function and use of the GP more clearly and relearn how their professional role fitted in with the rest of their lives.

The group offered a space to work through a lot of pent-up feelings and widened and deepened their understanding of the themes which surfaced during the pilot phase of the project. In the group the GPs were able to let go of the predominantly resentful relationships within the NHS; they found real co-operative relationships in the group, internalised these and transferred them as coping skills into their own primary care context. The groups were designed to offer a transitional space which could foster mutual support and help each doctor gain rather than lose credibility with their peers. They shifted the use of the self in a relationship from a defensive stance and began to present their true and whole self irrespective of context and hidden agendas.

The main outcome of year 1 was a reconstruction of the GPs' professional identity in the light of current realities in primary care. The other major achievement of the group was to enable most of its members to separate from the role of helpless victim and recover the leader within capable of coping with a lot of uncertainty. There is no real way of predicting how long some people will take to accept and implement the latest reform. PCG leaders should therefore work with the grain of the group, not against it.

As a supervisor I tried to help these GPs cope better with the changes in primary care by opening the psychological boundary between the worlds of the doctor and the health manager. It was also important to me to revisit the taken-for-granted relationship between doctor and patient and explore how the one-to-one and the group dimensions related. In the unconscious mind of a GP the patient is the object of death, illness and misfortune and the doctor is in a state of health, eternal youth and immortality. Anton Obholzer (Obholzer and Roberts, 1994) has pointed out that there is a parallel between psychic processes in the individual and institutions. He says that the unconscious mind does not have a concept of health; instead it has a deep sense of death. To defend against our constant anxiety about mortality we develop psychological defence mechanisms. One of these is to pervert the health service in our minds into a keep-death-at-bay service. From a psychic point of view, therefore, doctors in a PCG and their separate primary care teams are a continuation-of-life service. In our predominantly narcissistic age primary care is expected to keep all the patients ageless and invulnerable and protect them from any change to the self-ideal of the designer healthy person (Lasch, 1979).

Politicians and their servants in the health bureaucracy are part of the pleasing business and have ended up setting fantastic targets for health promotion and the reduction of certain mental illnesses. These targets are met by primary care workers through resentful compliance and the falsification of statistics. These high expectations amount to a form of magical thinking within primary care and have unconsciously increased the pressure on the doctor to be the magician and priest substitute. In defence against this increased psychic pressure, the doctors in this group seemed to have withdrawn into a pre-Balint and very Cartesian model of medicine. In their view of general practice only the body counted and the anxiety-containing and psychological function of general practice was neglected. In consequence, the real skills of a GP were undervalued.

The more PCGs collude with setting unrealistic health targets, the more they will be in danger of failing. If they succumb, PCGs will risk setting up a version of the fatal collusion between doctor and problem patient when they fool each other into believing that they can prevent increased discomfort and pain and the inevitability of death. Ironically, the attempt to withdraw from the increasing chaos that walks through the surgery door into an idealised world of proper medicine increases the mayhem. Instead of making the consultation safer in a psychological sense, GPs are experienced as less caring and consequently they get swamped with even more anxiety from their problem patients. Patients living in an overly health-conscious society increasingly use the doctor as a protection against the dangers of living and the certainty of death. Doctors respond to the pressures of perfectionism by colluding with the patient to prevent a discovery of their impotence and inability to really help. This collusion increases the risk of complaints and litigation. All these themes were brought into the group and people relearned the art of boundary setting and realised that they can't escape the unconscious wish of society to shield its members from death and misfortune.

The GPs in the group realised that relief from stress comes from learning that reality has to be accepted rather than fought and that a distinction must be made between what is changeable and what is not. When this is done then doctor, patient and staff member can start to inhabit a system of relationships based on what is 'do-able'. Paradoxically, they then achieve a degree of change and improve efficiency by staying in touch with the sheer difficulty involved in succeeding in primary care. The protection against this wishful thinking lies in recovering the doctor's real professional self. Only self-confident GPs can stop colluding with the false ideals and expectations put upon them by politicians, managers and patients. Resisting magical thinking puts GPs back into the place where they have always been – in charge of primary care.

Year 2: working through the trauma of sadomasochistic training

The year 2 group revealed how the traumatic training experience of young GPs catches up with them during the transition from early- to mid-career and profoundly influences their ability to deal with reforms such as the launch of PCGs. The group ended up re-enacting some of the socialisation traumas associated with medical school. The first trauma is that of them missing adolescence due to the pressures of school and meeting parental expectations; the second is the sadomasochistic training at medical school and students' submissive socialisation into their professional belonging group. These experiences produce a paradox in that doctors appear capable of working in a co-operative mode in polite and idealistic teams but, underneath, they are individualistic, detached and controlling: the very opposite of a person with a propensity for PCG and multidisciplinary team membership.

When something has been experienced as a trauma it can't be worked through verbally, it has to be re-enacted. Only when the elements of the original trauma have been acted out in the safe environment of a supervision group can verbalisation and reflection begin. As the group members were all GPs in their early to middle 30s, the group took on the feel of an adolescent peer group. There was a lot of jostling for power and status between the men and women. The more unconscious members of the group spent a lot of time testing the boundaries and the integrity of the authority figures. In an adolescent peer group the unconscious leaders try to assuage their guilt for wanting symbolically to kill off the parents by splitting the parents into one good one and one bad one. The senior lecturer from the medical school became the good parent outside the group, the group analyst became the hated object in the group. Both the loved and hated parental objects were required by the adolescent group to define their own adult personalities – the one to identify with, the other to separate from. The process works best if the parents cotton on to the splitting process, reunite and form a holding alliance in which the feeling associated with moving from dependence to independence and interdependence can be owned, shared and discussed.

On two occasions the ambivalence about interdependence, group membership and authority was acted out. One group member shared important information only with the senior lecturer from the medical school and swore this person to secrecy. The secret was eventually revealed through a hunch I had. His naming of the secret in the group had two quite powerful effects. The senior lecturer was unburdened and empowered to function as a fully adult member of the group while the group member lost all trust in the group and used a change in partnership as a way to leave. One could simply locate the problem in the personal ambivalence of this GP towards all groups or in the failure of the group analyst to hold this person in the group. Both these aspects have a bearing on the story but there is also a group dimension to be considered. The ambivalence of this GP embodied a deeper psychic conflict in each GP between the idealised team approach to general medicine and the denigrated single-hander method. Inside each GP there is a single-hander waiting to get out and it is clear from the work in the group that single-handers have a lot of strengths which need to be integrated in a group approach to primary care. Equally, it became clear that groups in primary care do not just offer benefits but also add considerable stress to the lives of each GP within a partnership. In PCGs it has to be possible to integrate the single-hander and partnership approach; a space must be made for individuality and communality in the same group.

The other significant event in this group involved boundary and authority testing. I had conducted individual assessment interviews with a control group during year 2 which involved seeing some of the partners of the GPs in the group. After one group session, which dealt with a malfunctioning partnership, I felt compelled to give some advice to one of the group members who seemed distressed after the group had ended. She felt betrayed by this approach as I was seemingly breaking confidentiality about her partner in the control group. The group member called an extraordinary meeting to explore the possibility of leaving the group, having the group stopped or getting a new group leader. Again, the senior lecturer was put in the role of the good mother, the conductor in the dock as the bad father. The group member occupied the position of the innocent victim in charge of morality and order.

By now the group had developed a sufficiently strong matrix to hold and contain the anxiety and bring the unbearable feelings back into the group. The group analysed how this doctor repeatedly ended up in the public prosecutor role in partner groups and how the group analyst got sucked into an overenthusiastic helper role. The split symbolised one of the double binds which doctors have to live out: the carer with limitless supplies of concern and no boundaries, and the strict and consistent upholder of high standards of public morality. During the working though of this conflict in the group it became possible to reown the fact that general practice is work at the boundary and involves lots of imperfect compromises. The incident was also seen as a re-enactment of little acts of betrayal and rule bending that occur in all partner groups and help the practice to function.

The outcomes of year 2 were significant and varied. Several group members restructured their careers in line with their own abilities and one took over the senior partner role. Several women GPs decided to have babies during the year and moved from feeling that they had to choose between career and family to finding a way of combining the two. At least three out of the 12 became leaders of PCG pilots and formed a self-help group which continued to meet after their supervision group had ended. When the group felt more secure its members rediscovered how their sense of self-worth had been a product of the quality of their relationships with mother, father, siblings and medical teachers. This recognition allowed the group to separate the true and false selves of most of its members. When this work was done some GPs realised consciously that they had reached the boundary of a transitional stage in their lives which involves a mourning-liberation process (Pollock, 1980). The group had to let go of youth and its unattainable ideals. When they had accomplished this, they could accept reality in a new way.

Year 3: dealing with New Labour and primary care pilot groups

The third year of the project continued the underlying themes of all three supervision groups: the GPs' desire to use their feelings as well as their intellect, to take charge of and balance their lives and accept responsibility for further reform in the primary care sector. The first year had been about reworking the past, accepting the loss of a Golden Age and facing a new government and its ideas about primary care. The second year had struggled to move from late adolescence into full maturity and had integrated home and work more successfully. The third year met with New Labour in power abolishing fundholding and introducing PCGs.

Balint argued that medical schools in the 1950s taught one-person medicine with the doctor as the subject in charge and the patient the object of the treatment. His work helped to establish two-person medicine as standard practice in medical schools and helped us see the doctor–patient relationship as an interactive process. The third year of the project was facing up to locality commissioning and thereby a group matrix model of medicine. The Labour Party's reform of primary care takes multidisciplinary teams to their logical conclusion and forces GPs to develop the ability to perceive themselves as an interdependent figure in a matrix organisation. The most important elements of this primary care matrix are the doctor–patient relationship, doctor–staff relationship, doctor–PCG link and doctor–secondary and tertiary sector partnerships. It was becoming clear during the third year that the practise of modern medicine really is dependent on the acquisition of group skills and the ability to network on various levels of the system.

The relationship of each GP to the group changed from one of fear to one of appreciation shortly after the reforms were announced in Parliament. Current fashion in primary care would say that the Balint model is redundant but it should be remembered that the Balint group was a sophisticated instrument for measuring the quality of care provided by GPs long before audit and evidence-based medicine became fashionable. As a facilitator I tried to retain the idea that the group is a sensitive instrument for research into general practice. I trusted the group process to dramatise the real issues in primary care during the supervision sessions and thereby discovered the real and quite distinct training and development needs of each year group. I would do the same if such groups were institutionalised as part of a support package designed to ensure the success of PCGs.

By opening the boundary between the case presentation and the rest of the doctors' world I found that the Balint model gets stuck in a dyadic view of the world. I felt the need to widen the parameters of the group to a triadic and matrix view. If doctors are to cope with the medical, managerial, political and personal demands in a PCG they must have the capacity to accomplish in a group setting what they used to do in a dyadic relationship. Balint's thinking on groups derives from Freud, Klein and Bion. Freud reduced the relationship of the individual and the rest of the group to a dyadic scene of one mentally merged group and its unconsciously chosen father or mother figure. The Kleinians and the British School of Psychoanalysis perceive the group as a merged parental figure facing the person within it who tries to retain a sense of self and an intact professional identity. The Tavistock model claims that in a group the early relationship between mother and child gets re-enacted. Klein (1963) argued that any person who enters a group experiences a loss of sanity, rationality and ego strength. To defend against the resultant fear of disintegration, group members resort to psychological defences which function to reduce anxiety and maximise safety. Her pupil Bion (1961) identified three basic defences against the fear of being swallowed up by the group and losing any sense of self.

For most of one term the third year practised living through Bion's basic assumption positions in defence against yet more change brought in by the Blair government. The group avoided frank and honest exchanges by talking the present out of court and focusing instead on the past and the future. Rather than use the open space of the group to share current difficulties in their general practice, the shame attached to being imperfect was avoided by talking a lot about outsiders and the wicked, GP-hating politicians. The group used the politicians to avoid confronting one of its members who was perceived by the others as group-destructive and overly needy. Instead of facing the conflict with the rebellious adolescent and needy baby within and working these uncomfortable feelings through, the group allowed this person to take over the leadership in the heart-sink patient role. The consequence of this act of submission was that the group had a sidelined conductor, an inappropriate leader and an infantilised and helpless membership. I expect such a scene will be repeated in all those PCGs containing doctors with borderline personalities who cannot be contained or confronted by any of the leaders or the group.

If one adopted the classic dyadic model of looking at such a group situation (based on the analyst–analysand relationship), the problem would be located in the pathology of the individual who is acting out his or her anxiety in order to defend against the fear of being destroyed by the group. Alternatively, the problem could be located in the failure of the group to assert itself and in the failings of the group conductor. In my view everyone is involved in the dramatisation of a deeper truth which relates to the underlying fear in the group about the current mental trap of yet another primary care reform which everyone in the group faces with equal dread. Everyone (including the person who acted out the disturbance) used everyone else in the group to give expression to what could not yet be faced and put into words.

The group was living a phenomenon described by Christopher Bolas (1994) as the psychoanalysis of the 'unthought known'. By this, he meant that our unconscious often knows of an imminent destiny which our conscious mind is not acknowledging. Looked at in this way, the individual fighting for psychological survival and against internal fragmentation uses the group to defend against feelings and ideas which are better kept unconscious and which amount to the fear of not having enough inner strength for attachment to a group. The problematic individual in this group was, at a very deep and preverbal level, in touch with everyone's fear of annihilation through the establishment of PCGs. The person sensed the lack of safety and re-enacted an experience of inadequate mothering and loss of trust in authority figures in the group. The expression of this projected anxiety met the fears of the other GPs who felt that the next reform would change their professional sense of self beyond recognition and that no single-hander or partnership would survive in a desirable form. Like the anxious individual, the group also doubted whether it had the mental strength to live through yet another separation and attachment experience without loss of control and sanity.

A group can easily be taken over by a preverbal leader who attacks the thinking space in the group by outpourings of anger and resentment. Such a leader is accepted by the group when its members feel like retreating into a state of sulky silence, wish to attack the value of the meeting and resent what the perceived parent figures are up to. As the majority in this group had opted for the role of the Greek chorus and left the heroes (group conductor and unconsciously chosen antileader) to battle it out, it took many sessions before the most unconscious parts of the group's defences against reality surfaced. The example shows that the Balint dictum to exclude transference and countertransference issues from support groups with GPs cannot be maintained in the current context as the anxiety engendered by the primary care reforms produces borderline rather than neurotic forms of communication. This conclusion has a direct bearing on PCGs. These groups will also have the feel of a paranoid-schizoid group in which people deal with their ambivalence about membership being in the group through action rather than dialogue. Communication will take the form of absenteeism, lateness, sabotage of the agenda, rivalry and attacks on the leadership and the value of the group itself.

Conclusions: the added value of supervision groups

Ways of seeing among GPs

All three years unconsciously reproduced the Balint approach in that they dealt with every problem discussed in a doctor–patient framework. Whoever spoke first got diagnosed, labelled and fixed with a treatment plan. Self-psychology is a new branch of psychoanalysis which has altered the importance of childhood for our development. Kohut (1971) has argued that we must review our sense of self throughout life. Therapy and supervision consist of helping people adjust their self-ideal in the light of change in the internal and external world.

By this definition, the work in the Bolingbroke groups had desirable therapeutic outcomes. Self-therapy became necessary for these GPs because well-imprinted internal and biographically based methods of dealing with the outside world no longer seemed to work and caused symptoms of mental distress. By working in an experiential group, the GPs learnt to integrate the dyadic model of relating with one based on a group matrix. In that process they recovered their social selves and re-created their professional identity in such a way that the conflict between their own need to be independent and the need of the group to have its members be dependent could be tolerated without undue stress.

A new sense of self and professional identity is needed for GPs

All the GPs participating in this project were stressed out and needed new self-objects to identify with and hold in mind to give them the strength to face a primary care world which had been restructured yet again. The group members and the conductor of the group made these adjusted 'self-objects' available for identification and introjection for 90 minutes every week and offered each participant a chance to rearrange their inner matrix of relationships. Since this new inner matrix was based on a group model and went beyond the dyadic doctor–patient framework, it equipped these GPs for the world of PCGs. Yalom (1980) has pointed out that periodic adjustments in the self are linked to stages in the life cycle; this implies a movement towards maturation and each transition represents a preparation for death. We all know about these facts of life but we don't want to think about them. Consequently, we make this knowledge unconscious and start building up pretend scenarios, a false world which protects us from the inevitability of change and death.

Change is linked symbolically with death in the mind

In the unconscious mind change is linked with death and the two become interchangeable. Successfully implementing a fundamental primary care reform or a treatment plan for a patient requires a mature attitude towards the mortality of all things human – be it the body, the mind or an institution. Yalom (1980) wrote that we tend to defend against our underlying anxiety about death through compulsive heroism, workaholism and narcissism. These are indeed the symptoms of GPs in a state of stress and in danger of burn-out.

All three supervision groups spent a considerable time analysing the impact of death on their medical work. In year 3 the theme of death had a particular poignancy because the new reforms were anticipated as a form of death threat by the single-handers. At a personal level, several people had lost their partners and one group member had witnessed a terrorist attack in the Middle East in which many people had died. These very deep and serious reflections in the group had practical results. The group moved from defending against loss of control by recognising that communication, like fate, is not controllable. PCGs are an attempt to overcome the tribal warfare between competing GPs in a geographical area and between them as a group and the secondary care sector and health authority. This change is experienced as an attack on the symbolic order which governs the primary care universe. It is one thing for a government to design a reform of the primary care sector; it is another for the new vision to be accepted. The process of implementation will depend on a reconstruction of the symbolic universe inhabited by GPs and others in the NHS. Before anything is translated into practice, those affected by the new reform will have to negotiate the shared and divergent meanings of the change for them and how it can be squared unconsciously with their inner ability to live with interdependence with other subgroups within primary care.

Sacred medicine and profane politics in primary care

According to Wittgenstein, meaning is found through dialogue in a group context where people connect with the help of a shared language and the language games they have learnt throughout life. He showed how language games go beyond mere words and become a way of life. Doctors learn their language games at medical school and the language tools they are given to think with are proving inadequate in the face of the complex changes in primary care. Put stereotypically, doctors are socialised into a language game which distinguishes medicine and politics. Medicine is scientific and rational, politics is cultural and irrational. The reforms have made a nonsense of this split universe consisting of a pure and good half and a dirty and bad half. In the third year the group worked to re-establish medicine conceptually as a cultural and political as well as a biological and mental field.

The boundary between the sacred nature of medicine and science and the profane field of culture and politics had to be opened by these GPs before they could enter a PCG. When they allowed themselves to think about the link between primary care and politics, they could become active citizens and cope with the fact that they were in charge not only of bodily symptoms but also of social relations, political relations, economic factors and psychological phenomena. The groups became a transitional space for training in PCGs and through this work its members overcame their fear of pollution by getting involved with something which could be seen as political, self-seeking and non-altruistic. The segregated parts of the primary care cosmology could finally be integrated in the minds of most of these GPs to form a new medical self-object which was no longer a simple mirror of innocent natural phenomena but embraced the idea of medicine as a culturally constructed practice (Bourdieu, 1977).

Group stability and order depend on how we categorise the world

The anthropologist Edmund Leach (1986) showed how all humans and all groups need a sense of social order. Emotional stability depends on how we categorise and structure our worlds linguistically and conceptually. Order is accomplished through the telling of myths, the observation of taboos, adherence to binary thought and language patterns and the performance of rituals. At the core of the current primary care world is the myth of equality and the ritual of the multidisciplinary team meeting. Unconsciously, I would think, this model of being in a meeting has been transferred into the PCGs which are up and running. From a political point of view, this idealised and mythologised practice of working in teams mirrors the political goals of the 1960s protest movement which looked for communal and non-hierarchical forms of producing, relating and living. This middle-aged generation is now in power and our current national and local politics are shaped by their myths.

From a group analytic point of view the idealised and homogeneous team myth is a defence against the need of every group for structure, hierarchy, role differentiation and leadership. It can be interpreted as a flight from reality and autonomy into dependency where the team becomes a mother who protects the children from the Oedipal conflict with the authority figure(s). From this perspective cohesive teams are bound to end up as inward looking, preoccupied with envy prevention and not focused on the job of serving patients. The same will happen to PCGs if they adopt an overidealistic creation myth and impose an overly flat model of structuring the group and its business.

Edmund Leach argued that human beings need to know that they naturally belong to one species and that they are culturally different from each other. The meaning of cultural diversity and human unity is that equality is a fantasy that stands in the face of evolutionary and historical reality. We need the simultaneous thought of people like us and people not like us and we want to know who we are, who we are not, who they are and who they are not. Kinship is the basic model enabling us to find the common and differentiating element between us. The three-generation hierarchy lies at the core of all human groups and a modified form of the three-generation model within an extended family system will best serve as the underlying principle for differentiation and structuration within primary care groupings.

Moral panic and the setting of boundaries

Group boundaries and structuring devices like roles and hierarchies give us a sense of order in an otherwise chaotic and amoral universe.

Against this background, social anthropologists believe that change is a moral event which implies a rupture in the moral order of the world as we know it. This invokes feelings of moral panic, a search for salvation, persecution, scapegoating and rescue through heroes who easily become sacrificial lambs.

The third year of the LIZEI project unconsciously explored these archetypal cultural metaphors. The group faced up to the mature task of differentiating those who were expected to be the winners and losers in the new PCGs. When the group engaged in this difficult task it became possible to see that each person could not alter the reality of the latest reform but could now choose to become a perpetrator, victim or bystander. Those who decided that they were going to become active citizens and not take this reform lying down were the ones who accepted that primary care had become politicised.

It was the famous sociologist of a previous generation, Max Weber (1963), who put forward the thesis that each civilisation is organised around a 'soteriological vision' by which he meant ideas about suffering and how they are transcended to achieve salvation. In a secularised society like ours, this becomes even more important as religion is no longer the only regulator of what is right and wrong. The vacuum left by religion is filled partly with health and health promotion. The search for immortality and the body-beautiful and the avoidance of pain has become the regulator of moral codes. Doctors in our culture are given the role of the high priests who decide who belongs to 'us'; the healthy, upright citizens, and who to 'them'; the deviant, the unnecessarily ill and excluded people.

Working with this material in the group exposed the collusion of the doctors with the fantasy. They mirrored such thoughts by splitting patients into goodies and baddies and punishing themselves if they could not live up to the projected ideal of the good GP. The good GP is the one capable of coping with all the problems that walk through the door and able to please everyone equally. The bad GP is the one who is unknowing, helpless and powerless in the face of fate. It was by taking their political and professional fate back into their own hands, by participating in the PCG pilots and by turning the Bolingbroke group into a self-help forum that these GPs recovered their ability to set boundaries for patients. By exchanging their experience of stress in primary care, they recovered a sense of their own need and started the work of disabusing society and their clientele of their unrealistic expectations of primary care. PCGs, if they can be made to work, put GPs back into a position of power where they can renegotiate the social contract between themselves, the government and the patients. Indirectly, PCGs could help society adopt an adjusted soteriological vision, a vision which is less demanding of the magical powers of the GP and expects, instead, the patient to be more autonomous and grown up.

Letting go of an overidealised medical role

Being a mature GP in a PCG context requires the replacement of an exclusive and overidealised medical role with a role set which includes patient care, staff management and liaison with the system. The research aim for the group analyst in the LIZEI team was to test the group analytic model which does not focus exclusively on the doctor–patient relationship. In the groups doctors were encouraged to explore their shattered professional identity. The Balint focus on the doctor–patient relationship as the key to solving primary care problems was appropriate until the 1970s when the doctor felt looked after by the staff and was respected by the patients. In the current context no GP will be able to manage the job without leadership skills, the ability to be in a group and business know-how. PCG members will be in a better position to shape the reform and use it to get their own needs met if they find a way of overcoming the split between sacred clinical work and profane management. By integrating both activities in an overall conception of the total workload, PCG members and their PHCTs can begin to relate in a resentment-free way and unlock enough internal resources to take more collective responsibility.

The mindset needed to make primary care groups work

I am arguing for a different mindset in primary care, a paradigm shift. Marcel Proust is reputed to have said that rather than give him colonies and new worlds to look at, he would be happier if he were given a new pair of eyes with which to view the world. So, in the end, I think the way we look at a reform process will greatly influence how we survive the reform. The key question is whether we can use the crisis to reinvent ourselves or whether we will withdraw further into a sense of social isolation and failure.

Summary

Growth and development could result if PCGs accept the following points.

- A perspective on groups which allows for conscious as well as unconscious processes.
- An assessment of the change process which caters for progress as well as regression and takes heed of the psychological time and space dimension.
- The introduction and financing of supervision and learning groups as a way of enhancing levels of competence.
- Medical leadership on the clinical, managerial and group process levels.
- A view of leadership which accepts the need for it and regards the leader as situationally bound in a group.
- A way of turning reviews and audits into learning experiences rather than moral crusades and enforcement activities.
- A shift in the culture away from control and planning towards process, trial and error and learning from experience.

- Adopting a consultative leadership style.
- Accepting that politics and medicine are now as integrated as management and medicine.
- Testing of reality through a change model which is based on loss, separation, mourning, reparation and re-creation.

MODEL 1 GPs	MODEL 2 MULTIDISCIPLINARY TEAM MEMBERS
Target group	*Target group*
• GPs who are underperforming • GPs in need of support • GPs who want refreshment • GPs who want to spend PGE on experiential learning	• Key members of PHCTs who are underperforming, in need of support and who want to spend their personal and professional development time on experiential learning
Ideal group composition	*Ideal group composition*
• Heterogeneous, a mixture of the above	• Heterogeneous, a mixture of professionals • Homogeneous consisting of groups who are not doctors
Time needed	*Time needed*
• Five PGE days over one year	• Five days over one year
Accreditation	*Accreditation*
• Dean of PGE	• Dean of PGE
Recruitment	*Recruitment*
• Health authority • Self-referral • PCG/PCT education lead • PHCT	• Health authority • Self-referral • PCG/PCT education lead • PHCT
Programme	*Programme*
Day 1 + 4 • 3 EXPERIENTIAL GROUPS • 1 STRUCTURED WORK SHOP SESSION	Day 1 + 4 • 3 EXPERIENTIAL GROUPS • 1 STRUCTURED WORK SHOP SESSION
Day 2 + 3 • 2 EXPERIENTIAL GROUPS • 2 STRUCTURED WORK SHOP SESSIONS	Day 2 + 3 • 2 EXPERIENTIAL GROUPS • 2 STRUCTURED WORK SHOP SESSIONS
Day 5 • Coaching and support of individuals as needed	Day 5 • Coaching and support of individuals as needed

Figure 6.1: Continuing medical education model of personal and professional development, based on experiential learning.

CHAPTER SEVEN

A group analytic view of organisational development

The mid-life crisis of primary care

Most people live a paradox: their lives could be defined as a series of change events leading to the one thing which is absolutely certain – death. Yet most of us live life in such a way that we deny death and pretend that security, prosperity and health are forever. Many organisations have behaved in the same way. Until, that is, the advent of the six forces which began to change the form and self-perception of most organisations, including the primary care sector, over the last two decades. These forces, which have induced a kind of mid-life crisis in most organisations, were:

- globalisation and its twin, new public management
- customer power
- investor power
- information technology
- re-engineering
- the drive towards fewer layers of management.

The message has been of a double-bind nature: be more responsible, have less control.

During a mid-life crisis a person and an organisation have to find time and space to think, to take stock and rediscover a direction and identity. Group analytic sessions in the form of small self-experience groups, modified action learning groups or whole system meetings in large groups provide such a space for reflection and readjustment. In such a space, protected by a time boundary and facilitated by a skilled group analyst, people can rebuild themselves sufficiently to start recovering the losses incurred during change management programmes.

The exploration of unconscious processes in a group brings us to our senses. In the end, I would argue that the thrust of the current health reform is based on a denial. We pour all our energies into continuous improvement management in order to avoid the certainty that we have an ageing population that will not be made healthier but is more likely to need care for chronic conditions. The government could do with some group analysis to explore its fear of facing openly and honestly whether people are prepared to pay more in taxes to receive better healthcare. Instead of finding ways of offering patients real medical choices and reducing waiting lists and bureaucracy, politicians adopt 'patient empowerment' schemes which, from a psychoanalytic point of view, overburden the patient with decisions when they need care and a trusting relationship with their doctor.

The sociologist Anthony Giddens (1999) has argued that we are in the midst of a revolution that is inadequately described as globalisation. What is really going on, he says, no one really knows. We are able to collect some of the symptoms and diagnose the implications for each of us. The main personal consequence is that we get 'dis-embedded' from our learnt notions of social identity, social time and social space. These constructed notions, including our vocational identities, are now as much subject to fluctuation and rebranding as the organisation which serves as a belonging group for many of us and lends us an identity. The professional and private selves have become a 'reflexive project'. This means that we have to imagine, like idealist philosophers have done, that the world does not objectively exist out there in social structures or forms of professional organisation but is held in our minds. Reality is our perception of it; the world only exists if we say it does. Social reality is made by meeting in social situations and re-creating and reconstructing the meaning of this social reality through these encounters in everyday life.

So, when we talk of our sense of self, our sense of being a professional and a PCG member, we simply say something about our attempts to construct meanings in everyday life which help us survive the chaos which is normality. There is no fixed meaning attached to these social structures 'out there' or our inner working models of identity – they are continuously remade in face-to-face meetings. Globalisation has meant that the illusion that we can gain an identity from our culture is gone. We have to revise our ideas of self, of profession and of role as we go along and adapt them in a Darwinian way to a fast-changing environment characterised by increasing risk and uncertainty. The social game we are globally caught up in is one of survival, adaptation and extinction.

Change is accomplished through mourning

Many psychoanalysts and group analysts in the clinical setting have learnt that a person who can mourn the loss of youth and face mortality can disengage from destructive competition with imaginary enemies and concentrate on being creative, productive and mature. Organisations, including the NHS and its primary care sector, are currently in a similar position. Success doesn't necessarily come from driving down your competitor's prices or opposing the system but lies in focusing on releasing the creative synergies in the existing organisation and forming partnerships with other players in the same market or service sector in order to minimise the effects of uncertainty and chaos. The skills to manage in such a context are new and different; they centre around the mastery of compromise and reconciliation of conflict.

Modern GPs and practice managers need to create an organisational atmosphere in which people can become more adaptive, creative and mature. The experiential space of a group analytic session allows such qualities and skills to be explored in relation to real problems in the organisation. Permanent adaptation, relearning and reaccreditation are becoming institutionalised in all professions. I don't see how GPs can resist retreating into an autistic bubble of defensive isolation if they do not have a safe space in which they can recover their senses, share their difficulties with like-minded sufferers and then move on to rehabilitate their lost sense of self and integrity. A supervision group offers such a reconnecting container.

Many modern managers and management consultants do not visualise clearly enough that each change involves a separation from something held dear and an attachment to something unknown and feared. To negotiate the transition from the old to the new, an organisation has to work through a process of mourning. When an organisation is unable to mourn its losses it will suffer from a reduced capacity to be innovative and energetic. Many change leaders are frightened to admit that the transition from the old to the new, from local to global involves both progress and regression. No matter how sophisticated the change management technique is, change is a stimulus to the few and a threat to the many.

Working with the shadow of the organisation

Primary care groups will be more likely to succeed if policymakers and groups can work with the shadow side of an organisation and make room for the unexpected to happen. It is not normal for a reform plan to be implemented in its intended form. Change management books often pretend that most people in an organisation are willing to change while a few resist and can be dismissed. My experience has taught me that the opposite holds true. The problem is how sometimes the few can help the many feel safe enough to separate from their fear of change and take the risk of embracing the new vision, organisational structure and method of production or service delivery. At other times the majority in the group is needed to stand up to the so-called change enthusiasts and protect them from their own method of dealing with the fear of change.

Change leaders themselves are often the most threatened by change but protect themselves from being found out by rushing into compliance with reform. Internally, they are in what Freud called the anal phase of development where the child is potty trained and learns to comply with the parents' wishes whilst 'retaining' the capacity for non-compliance. Through potty training we built up our internal models of sharing, holding on, asking, refusing; in short, the quality of that experience determines greatly how we relate to authority in ourselves and others. When we are asked to attach to a fundamental change we regress internally to this early stage of development and have to relive the memories of it before we can engage with the repeat of the performance. If we are asked to let go of the last reform and adopt the new one, we are internally asked to relinquish what we have previously been force-fed and adopt the unwanted food as a new diet. Not only are we asked to digest the new food properly but we are also meant to produce healthy and sufficient faeces for inspection. Only when the manager has run the right audit tests and found the system to be appropriately compliant will we be given the feedback that we have been a good girl or boy by the organisational parents.

I believe that the creation of group analytic spaces during a change programme to reflect on these experiences without the pressure to produce predetermined outcomes gives people the chance to stay in touch with the essential chaos of the implementation process. A skilfully facilitated group process will hold an organisation and its constituent parts together during a period of turbulence and stay in touch with the primary task of delivering the service whilst everyone gets sucked into obtaining charter marks or total quality accreditation. By offering a safe space for the expression of anxiety, fear and uncertainty, it becomes possible to manage change more consciously, predictably and rationally.

In a group analytic session members of an organisation can discover that they already possess the experience and skills needed to cope with a major restructuring of the organisation. Each group contains members who have had to deal with the impact of birth, marriage, divorce, illness and death in a family system. It is this knowledge that allows the facilitator to show the organisation and its managers that change is both ordinary and extraordinary and that each person, group and organisational system is well adapted to cope with its impact. The group analyst aims to help the group rediscover what it already knows and use this life experience to neutralise the threat of the unknown and move on from fear of the future to its mastery.

Group analysis was invented to remotivate officers and soldiers who had suffered shellshock during active service in World War II. Putting people in groups and letting them exchange their experiences helped them overcome their fear and reconnected them to the task of winning the war. What worked for them should also work with modern organisations dealing with the shock of globalisation of the world economy, the re-engineering of company structures or the introduction of the new public management processes of market testing and best value.

Group analysts believe that symptoms of 'dis-ease' and malfunction in a person or organisation are problems of 'unrelatedness' and communication. The purpose of group sessions over time is to find the connections which have been lost between team members, departments or the organisational members and their task. At another level, group sessions will reveal that we depend for maturity and effective performance on the integration of a sense of I, you and we and that performance suffers when one of these elements is experienced as overdemanding or depriving at the expense of another. For instance, if the mother company deals with its feared loss of importance during globalisation by denigrating its local satellites then the children that the organisation has spawned will never grow up and become successful because only mother is allowed to be perfect.

The added value of the group

Yet another level of group analytic work deals with the fact that humans are group animals and therefore depend on being in a relationship. Only when human beings feel connected enough can they become productive and creative. The group enables members of an organisation to revisit their social nature, their interdependence and independence with the inside and outside world. By enabling people to accept and work with their interdependence, group analysts hope to maximise constructive exchanges between people and reduce destructive, defensive and territorial behaviour which holds people, teams and organisations back from development and change. When sufficient basic trust between managers, teams, sections and the whole company has been established it becomes possible to share an overall workload, vision and strategy for the organisation because boundaries have stopped being barriers and become translucent.

Implicit in group analytic work is the idea that the group dimension of an organisation can add value to its performance. Matrix models of management have been idealised or denigrated for two decades. In practice they have often failed because they assume that groups are benevolent and that people have a preference for flat teams. It is thought that one has only to create group cohesion and send clear and transparent messages and all will be well. In reality things are more complex. Clinically speaking, cohesive teams are sick and engage in group-think. They will divert resources for their own perverse ends and forget about reality and the task. Healthy teams are able to become coherent about their own strengths and weaknesses, tolerate difference and accept interdependence; they also come to terms with the fact that managers and leaders are indispensable if a team or organisation is to function effectively. A well-functioning and trained group and its leader will not be afraid of contact with other groups within the organisation. They are happy to perceive the uncertain context of the world market or political environment in which they operate as a challenge and an opportunity to show their creative potential. The skills needed to create and maintain a healthy group need to be learnt through experience. I would argue that the open space in professionally facilitated group sessions should become an integral part of management and organisational development programmes.

Trusting the group

The group analytic technique turns the relationship between client and management consultant on its head and puts both of them back into the roles they should be occupying: the client in charge and the consultant the servant of the group. The group analytic approach to consultancy reveals that successful change depends on the creation of the group as a third partner in an alliance with the manager and the consultant. The group is the real added value during a process of transition. Most managers fear the group or don't trust it. Group analysts can show through their practice how it is possible to pacify the destructive forces within the group and redirect misdirected energy into creative and constructive channels. Once the synergy flows within the group, the organisation can be sure that planned change will result in actual implementation and results, provided it is not expected that outcomes and plans will be matching but will be a move in the right direction.

The group process will demonstrate repeatedly that developing plans, visions and strategies should be a means to an end, not an end in itself. When the whole organisation becomes committed to change, the plans will inevitably have to be adjusted and modified in the light of the experience of implementation. Comparing the difference between intent and outcome during group sessions designed to accompany the implementation process will enable the organisation to take another step towards building a culture where learning, knowledge exchange and continuous improvement are built into everyday life.

The group as a learning laboratory

Uncertainty, risk, chaos, globalisation, complexity and the learning organisation have been some of the keywords used by managers, consultants and academics over the last decade. There is agreement on the fact that these forces will shape the future organisation and determine what skills a modern manager needs. What is less clear is the best method for acquiring these new competencies and qualities. Group analytic sessions without a predetermined agenda allow participants to 'experiment' directly with uncertainty, chaos and complexity. The patterns of interaction and the flow of communication are never predictable in a group session and 'survival' depends on the use of life experience and trust in the other members of the organisation. People rediscover the ability to integrate thinking and feeling and use intuition and judgement to 'tame' the destructive forces and 'foster' the creative forces in the group through dialogue about common problems. Essentially, this is the task of the future manager and I see group sessions as the most appropriate training ground for acquiring these competencies. Regular group sessions can become a vehicle for the development of leaders, teams and the whole organisation whilst enhancing performance and growth.

The experience of mastering leadership skills in an open group session will develop the qualities organisations look for in their new managers. Such a person is a competent communicator and people manager who remains proactive in a situation when everyone else wants to be reactive, and fosters independence, interdependence and accountability. It follows that open group sessions offer managers and staff the opportunity to get away from divisive 'us' and 'them' relationships and help forge a real partnership designed to ensure the survival of the whole organisation and not just sectional interest groups. Open group sessions at regular intervals will enable an organisation to learn from its experience at the task and relationship levels. Attention to both these levels will enhance the ability of an organisation to be competitive and innovative and reduce the cost of change management in the medium and long term. Above all, group participants will be weaned from an overly individualistic perspective of performance and management and develop the capacity to put the group before the individual whilst not losing sight of their interdependence.

Mastering the future within the group

In a group analytic session organisational members and their managers can find ways of learning from each other and, through the exchange of practical experience, readjust the vision, strategy and operational procedures of the organisation in an ongoing process. Strategy becomes a conversation, a method of developing a flexible and adaptive shared mindset in the organisation, rather than a detached one-off during an away-day. Performance monitoring, knowledge management and learning become part of an ongoing process of reflection through self-experience, joint problem sharing and experiential learning.

Through dialogue in a group setting, over-risky and uncertain restructuring exercises can be avoided. Change builds on the culture which made the organisation survive and succeed in the first place. The facilitated group is an in-between space which can be likened to Charles Handy's 'empty raincoat' waiting to be filled with innovation, self-realisation and cultural meaning (Handy, 1994). The group provides a space in which organisational members can practise openness, direct communication and mutual help. By overcoming their fear of 'revealing' that they have a problem coping, individuals regain self-respect and credibility with their peers. They consciously own their resentment of clients, staff, partners and the changing external environment. Group members begin to acknowledge that they suffer jointly from change fatigue and feel the need to put themselves before the client, the problem or the boss. By exchanging common experiences of struggle and suffering, organisational members regain a degree of self-confidence and begin to reconstruct their professional identity and competence on an individual and group level. Subsequently, the energy devoted to defending against the seemingly endless and overwhelming demands starts to be redirected towards survival, re-creation and re-innovation.

In the group sessions I have described above, the GPs rediscovered 'real' relationships. They overcame their fear of conflict and disagreement and began to tackle the problems inside the group by telling each other what they liked and disliked, what they wanted to retain, what they wanted to change and what they were happy to negotiate about. Having expressed their repressed aggressive feelings towards each other and survived this potentially shaming experience, they internalised these new forms of relating as a good and bad person and were able to transfer the facility for open communication to their own organisations. The renewed authority with which they thought and spoke moved them and their teams on and many of their organisations appeared, on a follow-up visit, to be more modern and better working environments. A shift from a negative to a positive organisational dynamic had occurred, not by cleaning the organisation of all negative elements but by learning to perceive them as a normal part of reality and treating them as a potential source of energy.

The most important outcome of the weekly sessions was that most group members rethought and relaunched their careers in general practice. Being a 'mature' GP now requires the replacement of an exclusive and overidealised medical model with a role set which includes patient care, staff management and liaison with the system. In the group the non-measurable emotional side of the doctor, patient and staff personality was accepted as normal. The GPs learnt to deal with the paradox that the essence of the daily running of a primary care team is certainty whereas the essence of steering it towards the future is uncertainty. The groups demonstrated that the coping skills for dealing with the unknown, working in a team context and being an empathic leader are best learnt through 'supervision' in a professionally conducted group session.

An open group analytic session can be seen as a form of transition ritual which allows individuals, subgroups and the whole organisation to separate from the old forms of working and engage in a search for new forms of organising the work and competing in the marketplace. In a group it becomes easier for managers to close the gap between the intention to change and a successful implementation process by working with everyone on the performance and relationship levels simultaneously. Group sessions reveal how difficult it is for most people to hear the exhortation to change and grow up. Meeting face to face allows managers to connect structural changes with the people who have to translate the plan into operational reality and patient satisfaction.

The most effective way for a manager to become a leader during periods of uncertainty is by demonstrating an ability to be a listening but decisive and honest communicator. Clever visions do not necessarily inspire people to change but the feeling of being connected to a trustworthy leader and a committed group encourages people to let go and move on.

At the strategic level, it is time to recognise that a decade of top-down change management, based on grand structural re-engineering models, has not really improved the primary care system. It is time to give a bottom-up focus a chance and let PHCTs and PCGs find the change which will help them do the job better and trust that an accumulation of little changes will amount, in time, to a more significant improvement in service provision than grand change management schemes. In open group sessions within a PHCT and with PCGs, lasting relationships can be forged. Group analysts can help managers turn a group from being an obstacle to change into a safety net which gives the organisation the confidence to deal with an uncertain future and master it.

Table 7.1 Competing visions of how to 'manage' people within the NHS

Paradigm			
ECONOMICS	BEHAVIOURAL PSYCHOLOGY	SYSTEMS THEORY	GROUP ANALYSIS
Economic being	**Social being**	**Complex being**	**Group and social being**
• Efficiency • Task division • Scientific organisation • Admin focus • Cost control • Central authority • Discipline • Hierarchy • Standard work • Formal culture • Mass output	• Delegated • Self-realisation • Work groups • Flat power • Motivation through involvement • Enhanced work conditions • Trust • Consensus • Consultative • Informal	• Adaptation • Survival • Flexibility • Effective • Self-management • Devolved responsibility/power • Interacting internal/external world • Synergy search • Networking • Self-discipline • Maturity • Interdependent • Uncertainty • Risks • IT • Communication	• Matrix • Inter-dependence • Group process • Location of problem in everyone • Leader, follower and group one gestalt • Foundation matrix • Manage through group, with group, in the group • Manager as facilitator • Manager respects culture, process
Core idea	**Core idea**	**Core idea**	**Core idea**
DO-ABILITY	MOTIVATION	SELF-ORGANISATION	INTER-DEPENDENCE

Table 7.2 Organisational consultancy models for group and whole system development in primary care

PHCT	PCG	PCT
Methods • Individual coaching • Experiential learning groups • Problem-solving groups • Large groups	*Methods* • Individual coaching • Experiential learning groups • Problem-solving groups • Large groups	*Methods* • Individual coaching • Experiential learning groups • Problem-solving groups • Large groups
Intervention • 4 × ½ day with the whole team • 4 × ½ day with partners • 8 × ¼ day with uniprofessional groups • Individual coaching when desired or required • Fit in with existing meeting and planning schedules	*Intervention* • Large groups with the whole PCG or with CE, PCG board, management team and representatives selected by members • Experiential learning and action groups with management team • Experiential learning and action groups with PCG board • Individual coaching when desired or required for chief executive and educational lead • Length of time to be negotiated after diagnosis • Fit in with existing meeting and planning schedules	*Intervention* • Coaching of chief executive, educational lead • Development of PCT lay board, executive board and project groups through ongoing experiential learning and action groups • Large and small work groups with various stakeholders involved in the PCT to integrate the whole system and organisational culture so that it can hold members sufficiently to make PCTs work • Fit in with existing meeting and planning schedules
Outcome • More effective performance and service to patients • Accreditation • Dean of PGE • Referral • PHCT & PCG/PCT	*Outcome* • Effective performance of PCG • Referral • PCG/PCT/HA	*Outcome* • Successful institutionalisation and effective performance and service to patients

POSTSCRIPT

The support function of the group: relevance to education and training agendas for primary care groups/trusts

Simon Freeman

Introduction

The inevitable cycle of change within the NHS brings with it feelings of anxiety, dis-ease and uncertainty. The culture of the 'New NHS' forces us to grapple with new organisational structures, new models of care and new attempts to evaluate what we do. These changes are reflected in the new language we speak. Terms such as PCGs, PCTs, HImPs (health improvement programmes), PCIPs (primary care investment plans), clinical governance, revalidation and continuing professional development exemplify this. The concrete reality that reflects the change in language can be the extreme ends of a spectrum but is usually somewhere in between. Smoothly running organised structures working in collaboration contrast with administrative chaos hampered by individual agendas. Thick, indigestible, irrelevant and unread documents contrast with brief but meaningful analyses of local need and circumstances that lead to small but significant changes.

What was to have been a gradual evolution of PCGs over 10 years has rapidly developed into a lemming-like scramble to PCT status in a matter of two or three years. Politicians have not explicitly pushed for this but the political drive is certainly there. The anxiety generated by the thought of being left behind and missing out on the incentives given to those at the front of the queue means that many PCGs move more rapidly to PCT status than they would like. With any organisational change new skills need to be acquired to meet the needs of those that the organisation has a statutory duty to provide for. Are the strategies for education and training of the workforce in place?

Meanwhile GPs seek to redefine themselves in a world of greater public accountability where fitness to practise has to be demonstrated and can no longer be assumed. The prospect of revalidation creates its own anxieties on top of those that clinical governance brought. But maybe a clearer definition of what constitutes an acceptable level of performance and a re-evaluation of how to go about ensuring our ongoing education and professional development is welcomed by most. And long overdue.

How do GPs survive, reinvent and regenerate themselves and new models of primary care in the context of changes that are sold as opportunities but carry many hidden threats? In this chapter I offer some reflections on the lessons learnt from an educational group, 'the Bolingbroke Group', which seem very relevant. Particular emphasis is placed upon the support function of the group, which might most easily be developed within the context of an education and training agenda.

Clinical governance and revalidation

Issues relating to quality of care and public accountability have been highlighted as priority areas for PCGs/PCTs to address. Clinical governance is the 'framework through which NHS organisations are accountable for continuously improving the quality of their services and safeguarding high standards of care, by creating an environment in which excellence in clinical care will flourish' (DoH, 1998). In essence, PCGs/PCTs are being asked to demonstrate that they have a robust framework that will guarantee that these high standards are provided by the organisation as a whole and by the individuals working within it. The concept of continuing professional development of all PCG/PCT members with their own professional development plans is seen as fundamental to the success of this strategy.

Running in parallel with this organisational strategy is the belated attempt by the medical profession to demonstrate that it can be truly capable of regulating itself. Serious issues of poor performance and misconduct have called the concept of self-regulation into question. Now the various professional bodies that oversee the education, training and licensing of doctors are co-ordinating their efforts to set in place a process whereby doctors can be seen to demonstrate their fitness to practise. This process will be revalidation.

Meanwhile the government expresses a wider political and public view about the need to recognise and manage those doctors whose performance gives cause for concern in a consultation document *Supporting Doctors, Protecting Patients* (DoH, 1999). The failings of current approaches to identify and remedy poor clinical performance in the NHS are highlighted and new mechanisms are proposed. Few would argue with the principles embodied in the title of this consultation document but the proposals for the future seem to offer little in the way of support to doctors. Rather, a mechanistic approach that removes doctors from the context in which they may be underperforming eliminates opportunities to deal with organisational failings that may be contributing to, or resulting from, a doctor's poor performance. Scapegoating of the individual doctor, who may be a symptom of a much deeper malaise within the system, both at practice level and on a much wider organisational front, may undermine the aims and objectives of this initiative.

Continuing professional development and the group

The themes that are common to the principles of clinical governance, revalidation and structures and processes that will truly support and protect patients can be linked to those that are broadly accepted as best practice in medical education. The latter includes educational activity focused on everyday experience, reflective practice in the context of an audit/learning cycle, portfolio development, effective needs assessment, peer review, group-based learning and evaluation that will be both formative and summative. What emerges is a model of continuing professional development (CPD) that mirrors the structure and process embodied by the Bolingbroke Group.

In essence, the emerging model for CPD is one of peer review within the context of a group that is truly supportive. Only in an environment that feels safe will GPs, or members of any discipline, feel able to let their defences down and be honest about their own competence and performance. As will become clear in the review of the Bolingbroke Group, creating this environment and maintaining it is an active task and does not occur passively. If an educational group is to function optimally then skilled facilitation will be required. Facilitators in such a group need to pay attention to the matrix and transactions within this matrix if the group is to be supportive in such a way that excellence in clinical care can be defined, developed and allowed to flourish outside the group itself. The alternative is a group that at best ticks the boxes as each task is addressed and at worst is dysfunctional to the point of alienating its members as hierarchies emerge, subgroups plot, individuals become scapegoats and those most in need of support are too ashamed to ask the questions that deep down we all need to ask.

The Bolingbroke group demonstrated the rich rewards of having a group analyst to help disentangle the complex mix of agendas and anxieties that are brought to the group. Work at this level helped the individuals and group as a whole contextualise the educational tasks and thereby increased the likelihood that these would be undertaken successfully. When focusing on significant events within everyday experience, the group was able to undertake reflective practice at a deeper and more meaningful level than normally occurs within the context of an audit or educational cycle of change. Answers to reflective questions such as 'What am I doing?' and 'Why am I doing this?' start to put the behaviour of the individual in the context of psychodynamic driving forces, day-to-day social and political pressures, the large group that is the

NHS and the small groups that are our families, GP partners and primary care teams.

As an extreme example we might look at the question 'How do I deal with my murderous feelings toward my patient?' which would not be inappropriate in the context of a Balint group grappling with the dynamics of the doctor–patient relationship. Within the context of the Bolingbroke Group this question would have been extended to 'How do I deal with my murderous feelings toward my partner, my practice manager, my district nurse, my receptionist, my health visitor, etc.?' Individuals may become the scapegoats for feelings that are really directed at the wider system and its failings and so we should similarly ask 'How do I deal with my murderous feelings toward my local hospital, the Social Services department, the NHS, the BMA, the GMC – in fact all those individuals and organisations that have let me down or the 'mother' that has not been good enough?' In other words, if we fail to deal with our feelings, our projections in relation to individuals, groups and our partner organisations, we undermine our opportunities to undertake tasks in relation to them successfully. Hence, an educational group that is only task oriented may achieve some of its aims and objectives but at a deeper level real progress, real changes in attitudes and behaviour will not be brought about.

The Bolingbroke Group and lessons for primary care groups/trusts

The Bolingbroke Group was a group learning activity undertaken by GPs mainly in their mid-career. The group was established as part of the London Implementation Zone Educational Initiative (LIZEI) which sought to improve the retention, recruitment and refreshment of GPs in Inner London in the context of concerns about the quality of primary care being offered. While many of the activities that GPs undertook as part of LIZEI addressed their individual concerns, the Bolingbroke Group sought to confront the needs of the group as well as the individual. A fundamental principle underlying the activities of the group was that productive educational activity could only take place in an environment that was supportive, thereby allowing the problems of stress, low morale and burn-out that were being experienced by GPs to be explicitly addressed. Hence the group learning approach sought to address the failure of much postgraduate education to tackle these issues.

What lessons do the educational activities of three relatively small groups of GPs have that are relevant to the evolution and development of the much larger and more complex group that is the PCG/PCT – the latter being a large group that comprises members from a wide range of professional disciplines and also seeks actively to engage the public? If there are any lessons to be drawn they are those that relate to the support function of the group. Support of individuals, between individuals, of small groups within the larger group and of the PCG/PCT as a whole will be crucial to their success or failure. Perhaps more importantly, it will be crucial to the survival of individuals, whatever their stance in relation to the outcome of their PCG/PCT.

I acknowledge that it is simplistic to draw exact parallels between the Bolingbroke Group and a PCG/PCT but within this constraint I shall attempt to highlight some points for consideration. These may have relevance to the development of these organisations as a whole as well as to an education and training agenda.

The support function of the group

Fundamental to the success of the Bolingbroke Group were elements of support that were offered in a variety of ways. These enabled the group to develop a task-oriented approach to learning that addressed the needs of both the individual and the group. Support was offered to the following individuals and groups.

- GP members of the Bolingbroke Group.
- The practices that these GPs had left behind.
- The academic assistants providing support in the practices.
- The 'teaching team' facilitating the Bolingbroke Group.

Although I will concentrate on the support function of the Bolingbroke Group itself, it is worth noting that the support offered outside the group was a very important factor in the group's achievements. Parallels with the support needed to allow a PCG/PCT to function optimally are drawn.

The practices and organisations left behind

GPs were involved in the activities of the Bolingbroke Group for a full day a week over three 10-week terms during the course of a year. To leave practices unsupported for this period of time would have put an unacceptable burden on the GPs left behind and in the case of single-handed GPs would have made their involvement impossible. Locum cover was provided in these practices by academic assistants who were individually attached to practices, thereby providing a degree of continuity of care not normally present when locums are employed on an *ad hoc* basis.

Just as the Bolingbroke Group encouraged GPs to take time out of their day-to-day practice, the PCG/PCT places a similar demand on the time of its constituent members. GPs desert their surgeries, nurses their communities, Social Services representatives their departments, health authority members and lay members their respective organisations. They do this in the belief that their activities within the managerial and organisational structure of the PCG/PCT will serve a greater good and ultimately bring benefits to their patients, their clients, their own organisations, themselves and their colleagues.

But who will replace them in their normal role? Will colleagues cover for their absence, thereby increasing their own workload and creating feelings of resentment? Will patients understand why they are not as available as they were before? Or will these activists seek to take on the tasks within the PCG/PCT on top of all their normal duties? Will personal time be devoted to these activities at the expense of relationships within families and with friends? Is there a danger that the demands of the PCG/PCT will create stress and contribute to the premature burn-out of its active members? Does the reluctant and questioning member of the PCG/PCT who challenges the level of commitment required have an important message that needs to be heard?

Protected time in the form of proper support to the active

individuals and the colleagues and organisations they leave behind is vital. The Bolingbroke Group had the luxury of cover provided by academic assistants. PCGs/PCTs must identify how they are going to provide a similar high-quality level of cover and how this is to be resourced. Politicians must be made aware of the implications. At a time when recruitment and retention of GPs remains a major problem this message needs to be given a very high profile.

In addition, practices and member organisations of PCGs/PCTs must support their representatives who are actively engaged in the activities of the PCG/PCT. To encourage and fulfil this, PCGs/PCTs will have to communicate effectively with their members to ensure a clear understanding of the reasons for and potential benefits of the PCG/PCT. As the organisation evolves the corporate and inclusive nature of its activity will become increasingly apparent and should demonstrate the value of support at all levels.

Academic assistants and their equivalents in PCGs/PCTs

The academic assistants were employed by the Department of Primary Care at St George's Medical School. The majority of these were GPs who had recently completed their vocational training. Their contracts offered a combination of activities including sessions within the surgeries of the GPs attending the Bolingbroke Group, and opportunities to engage in research and teaching activities. Members of the Department of Primary Care offered them support. Inevitably issues arose in relation to the work undertaken in practices and opportunities to discuss and resolve these were provided.

PCGs/PCTs involve a wider range of professional groups and will have to evolve their own methods for providing the type of cover outlined above. In general practice, employment of salaried partners, assistants and retainers has enhanced the workforce but the locum doctor provides the bulk of cover for an absent doctor. Traditionally there has been a pool of doctors who have chosen not to become principals in general practice, who are between jobs or who have retired. Occasionally a locum will stay attached to practices for a length of time but more often than not practices are struggling to find adequate locum cover and it can be a case of employing whoever is available. Continuity of care becomes a problem and issues surrounding quality of care are difficult to tackle.

PCGs/PCTs have the opportunity to develop links with and support their locums. The Framework of Clinical Governance, with its emphasis on education and training, can support this. There is evidence to suggest that newly qualified GPs who form the bulk of the locum workforce would welcome a more supportive and structured approach to their continuing professional development (CPD). Attempts to integrate this group into the ethos of the PCG/PCT will encourage improvement in the continuity and quality of care provided. At a very simple level this might mean developing a pack for locums that contains information relating to guidelines used within the PCG/PCT. Invitations to attend and contribute to activity within the PCG/PCT will foster improved working relationships and also allow knowledge and information to flow from the locums into the PCG/PCT. The observations of the 'outsider' may teach us a great deal.

PCGs/PCTs also have the opportunity to explore alternative ways of providing services, as exemplified by PMS pilots that employ salaried GPs. These GPs will also need the support of their colleagues within the PCG/PCT if they are not to become isolated.

The nature of the GP workforce is rapidly changing. For example, increasing numbers of doctors wish to work part time or combine general practice with activities such as teaching or research, never mind a life outside work. This provides further opportunity for the PCG/PCT to consider how it can organise the workload in such a way that the employment opportunities become attractive to doctors who might otherwise leave general practice.

Developing and supporting the teaching team

The team that facilitated the activities of the Bolingbroke Group initially comprised a group analyst, a senior lecturer and a lecturer based in the Department of Primary Care, and three GPs from the locality. Over the three-year period this team evolved with increasing responsibility being borne by the local GPs, and the senior lecturer withdrawing to a more supervisory role. The group analyst worked with each of the three groups that were established at yearly intervals.

Before the group started meeting the senior lecturer facilitated the development of the teaching team. In particular, time was spent examining the theory and techniques employed in small group teaching. Throughout the duration of the group's life the teaching team spent time evaluating not only the progress of the group but also their own performance as teachers and facilitators. This process was primarily that of peer review. The support offered between the members of the teaching team enabled the ongoing development of teaching skills and the opportunity for them to address their individual and group needs as teachers. Given the dynamics of the groups, this was important to the development and maintenance of the group as a whole.

Are there parallels between the Bolingbroke teaching team and PCGs/PCTs? Educational leads will be identified and have an important role to play. Would it be stretching the analogy too far to suggest that there will be leads in all areas of PCG activity that imitate the role of the teaching team? Board members, for example? They will need to become leaders and facilitators within the PCG in relation to a wide range of activities. PCG/PCT chairs will have an over-riding responsibility while leads in areas such as clinical governance, HImPs, PCIPs and the like will help to develop a corporate responsibility within the PCG.

Chairs and board members in particular will be required to develop a new range of skills that combine an understanding of organisational development with financial acumen. Tasks previously undertaken and overseen by the management structure of the health authority will be devolved. The wider public health implications of decision making at practice level will become more explicit and the skills to commission services appropriately will be needed to fulfil the health needs of the PCG/PCT population.

Investment of time and energy in developing the relevant skills will be a necessary prerequisite for PCG/PCT boards and PCGs/PCTs as a whole to function effectively. Organisational development needs to be an active ongoing process that takes account of individuals coming and going, roles changing and the needs of the PCG/PCT changing over time. Already the writing on the wall suggests that evolution to PCT status is inevitable, no matter how hard the politicians seek to deny it. What will the educational needs of these organisations be?

Who will facilitate this process within the PCGs/PCTs? Health authorities have an obvious role to play but facilitation from outside sources will be important. PCGs/PCTs will be seeking guidance and facilitation both nationally and locally but, as with the Bolingbroke Group, mutual support within the PCG/PCT may help identify and develop skills that are already owned.

Education and training within the PCG/PCT

While the evolution of a PCG/PCT is in itself an educative process, within the PCG/PCT there will need to be a specific education and training agenda. Will PCGs/PCTs support the development of education and training at all levels and in all groups within the PCG/PCT? If so, who will the teachers be? How will their roles be defined? Who will they be responsible to? What support and resources will be made available? Who will facilitate their development?

National guidance clearly indicates that the development of a local education and training framework should be encouraged. In fact, continuing medical education in the form of CPD is seen as underpinning the development of an effective clinical governance framework. The PCIP should make specific reference to education and training. All members of a PCG/PCT are encouraged to develop their own continuing professional development plan (CPDP) that addresses not only their own needs but also the needs of the PCG/PCT.

Individuals who are identified to lead the development of the educational and training framework will themselves need support and facilitation. These individuals will span a range of disciplines and will need to develop a 'curriculum' that meets the needs of their own professional group as well as a multidisciplinary agenda.

A variety of models are already evolving. The sharing of ideas between these models and between PCGs/PCTs will be important. Opportunities for the members of education support teams to come together and also to meet with colleagues performing similar roles in other PCGs/PCTs will help move this agenda forward.

They will require the backing of the PCG/PCT board who in turn will need to understand and contribute to the 'curriculum' that a

PCG/PCT may develop. Facilitation and support from local educational consortia, medical schools, postgraduate deaneries and other relevant educational institutions will be important. These organisations can contribute to 'teaching the teachers' and facilitate the development of teaching skills within PCGs/PCTs.

Facilitation of the group

Facilitation and support were offered to individuals who joined the Bolingbroke Group by the teaching team even before the group itself started to meet. The process of recruitment, primarily undertaken by the local GPs in the teaching team, was a time-consuming activity that highlighted the difficulties of contacting and communicating with GPs. Once they had been contacted, the nature of the educational group and offer of protected time was explained. Interested GPs often expressed reluctance to join because they felt that they were deserting their patients or partners, while for others the process of negotiating time out of the practice was a difficult one. Whichever category group members fell into, the ongoing contact, support and encouragement of the teaching team members were vital to the recruitment process.

The initial meeting of each of the three groups formed was carefully planned bearing in mind the need to explore individuals' reasons for joining the group and providing an opportunity for anxieties to be explored. Time was spent explaining the background of the group and what individuals might expect to gain from it over the course of a year. Paired introductions facilitated the process of getting to know a little about each other on both a professional and a personal level.

Safety issues were raised very early in the discussion and led on to a degree of consensus around the rules that should operate in the group. Boundaries for sharing information together with the rules of confidentiality were discussed and agreed.

When group members were asked 'What do you want from this group?' common themes emerged, including:

- a chance to meet colleagues and share ideas
- support of a group
- time out of my practice

- clinical updates
- information about local services.

These 'wants' received concrete recognition when the group was asked to identify the topics that it wished to address in the task-oriented part of the day. In each of the three groups the same pattern emerged. Brainstorming generated topics for further discussion. The majority of these were clinical in nature. When asked to prioritise these as a group, using the nominal group technique, topics that addressed organisational and managerial issues, including stress reduction, together with personal development issues were strongly to the fore. It was as if individuals were unable to admit that they wished to address the problems of stress, low morale and burn-out but as a group with peer support, this was acceptable.

Perhaps the support and discussion within a group helped us to identify and admit to some of our educational 'needs' as opposed to our 'wants'. The evidence available indicates that individually we can be very poor at doing this.

Facilitation of the group is as relevant to a PCG/PCT as it is to a small educational group. Members of a PCG/PCT will need to be recruited to its culture. For the GP as independent contractor who has clung to his clinical freedom, the notion of adhering to guidelines and protocols agreed by the PCG/PCT may be anathema. Anxieties about the agenda of the PCG/PCT and the implications for individuals and their working practice will have to be explored. Ongoing support and encouragement will be a vital part of the process of active engagement.

Introductions and processes that lead to the building of relationships between individuals and member organisations will help overcome many of the fears that individuals may have and some of the barriers to progress that may be rooted in history. Effective communication will underpin this strategy. The communication network that is dominated by even bigger, and sometimes better, forms of IT will need to be counterbalanced by the immediacy of personal contact and communication. Only in this context will safety issues relating to the sharing of information, issues of confidentiality and the setting of boundaries be adequately explored. Effectively facilitated exploration of these issues will enable PCG/PCT members to build relationships rooted in mutual respect and trust that will allow real progress to be made when potentially difficult problems arise.

What will individual members want from their PCG/PCT? What will they have to offer? I suspect that the wants and needs will have many parallels with those of the Bolingbroke Group. Support in its various forms will be high on both lists.

Support from the group analyst

A regular feature of the Bolingbroke Group's activity was a 1½-hour session facilitated by a group analyst, Gerhard Wilke. Gerhard had previously worked with GPs and was familiar with many of the challenges that GPs face as clinicians and managers. Before the group was established he interviewed each group member and so had some insight into their individual circumstances and concerns.

The weekly session that he facilitated was an open forum to which group members could bring topics of any nature whatsoever. These were discussed and explored by the group and would often lead to the realisation of possible solutions. At the same time group members came to recognise the shared nature of many of the problems brought to the group and the value of seeking to deal with these as a group as well as individually.

The potential difficulty of groups being dominated by individuals who demonstrate an apparent confidence when working in a group setting is well recognised. However, it should be noted that the 'monopoliser' might be demonstrating their underlying anxiety when dominating the discussion within the group. This situation arose on occasion and highlighted the need for effective facilitation and support of the less vocal members.

While the group may have been able to address some of the issues that were presented without outside facilitation, we increasingly came to recognise the contribution that Gerhard made to our discussions. He brought with him a framework for examining and analysing topics that were primarily rooted in group analytic theory. This enabled the group to examine issues from a different perspective but perhaps more importantly, it prompted us to examine how we individually and as a group reacted to a variety of problems. Increasingly we came to recognise the powerful effect that our emotional and psychological responses had on the success or failure we experienced in dealing with particular problems.

In many ways this has obvious parallels with the ideas and theories developed by Balint and others since. However, these have mainly concentrated on the interaction between doctor and patient. The Bolingbroke Group examined these interactions but this form of analysis was developed to enable us to look at the interactions that occurred between ourselves, our partners (GPs) and other members of the PHCT. Taking this one step further, we explored our roles in the context of the health service and the wider social and political agenda. In so doing we were able to define some of the factors that contributed to feelings of stress, low morale and burn-out that we all felt to a lesser or greater extent. Similarly, we were able to identify those characteristics we possess as individuals and as a group that enabled us to take control and ownership of our destinies. The shared identity developed by the group was empowering and enabling to individuals when they went back to their practices to tackle some of the problems that they had previously regarded as insurmountable and insoluble.

Support from the group analyst in PCG/PCT? Is this such a far-fetched idea? There may well be times when individuals or groups within the structure of the PCG/PCT will welcome the insights of someone who is able to observe and analyse from a different perspective. This is relevant to the PCG/PCT as a whole and its individual subgroups – the board, practices, organisations such as Social Services, groups within the community trust, voluntary groups, public bodies and individuals. This becomes particularly relevant when individuals from different organisations with their different cultures start working together.

Educational groups within PCGs/PCTs may find sessions involving a group analyst helpful. Balint groups have served as models that have a proven role. The Bolingbroke Group provides a model that could be developed within a PCG/PCT.

The task-oriented sessions

These sessions were focused around the list of topics that the Bolingbroke Group identified and prioritised using the nominal group technique. From the outset, the teaching team sought to encourage the group to explore a variety of learning techniques.

Discussion within the large group, splitting into pairs and small groups, role play, the use of outside 'experts', research and presentations by group members were some of the methods that worked. Whichever method was used, the groups came to recognise the importance of sharing their own ideas, thoughts and experiences. This was a resource that became valued above all others.

Small group work altered the dynamic of the group and provided the opportunity for the less vocal members of the group to be heard. Working together on specific tasks and discovering more about each other was a powerful tool in building up mutual respect and understanding. The relationships created within the small groups helped build the confidence of the group members and would lead to active support and encouragement from their peers within the larger group.

When gaps appeared in our field of knowledge this naturally led to the generation of questions that group members endeavoured to answer themselves. Where this proved unfruitful, outside 'experts' were invited to join the group to discuss the questions. This produced a genuine discussion around topics where there was not necessarily any right or wrong answer. Again, peer support enabled individuals to admit to areas of ignorance. The realisation that our peers shared similar anxieties about acknowledging potential gaps in their knowledge and skill base enabled the group to work together in tackling these gaps. Similarly, the discovery that the invited experts did not know all the answers was reassuring. Their willingness to seek an answer to a problem in a collaborative process of research and discussion was mutually beneficial.

This was beautifully exemplified when one group constructed a questionnaire that addressed contentious issues in relation to maternity care. This was sent out to five local providers who generously responded. The range of answers to the questions asked was both remarkable and yet unsurprising. One respondent expressed surprise that we sought answers to these questions, even suggesting that all the answers were in the textbooks! The remainder demonstrated both wisdom and humility by indicating that they could not always offer definitive answers but suggested solutions on the basis of the best evidence available to them.

Drawing parallels with the task-oriented work of the Bolingbroke

Group can be done in relation to both educational issues and more general areas of work. Looking at the educational focus first, the opportunities for group learning within the PCG/PCT are obvious. The whole focus of the PCG/PCT is on a locality and the health needs of that population. The development of the HImP will highlight priorities of clinical need that will provide a natural focus for education in relation to clinical medicine. The PCIP will suggest areas of management and organisational activity that need to be addressed. Clinical governance will bring issues of quality to the fore. The clinical governance framework, National Service Frameworks and guidelines produced by the National Institute for Clinical Excellence (NICE) will provide a focus for learning that will need to be addressed by individuals, practices and the PCG as a whole. It will become obvious that the tasks being set by the national agenda will only be tackled successfully by a variety of unidisciplinary, multidisciplinary and interdisciplinary approaches.

CPDPs are expected to address the needs not only of individuals but also practices and the PCG/PCT as a whole. In the parlance of the group analyst, there is a coming together of the needs of the 'I' and the 'we'. Education and training activities are likely to be far more practice and locality based than in the past. This combined focus lends itself to multidisciplinary groups identifying learning needs, as opposed to wants, and prioritising areas of activity. For those who find the thought of this approach unhelpful, opportunity for individual mentoring by locally based peers could be developed. PCG/PCT-based training and education support teams could play a valuable role in facilitating this process. Drawing in appropriate experts and outside help will be focused on real need rather than the agenda and interests of the expert.

Already it is becoming apparent that the criteria for revalidation of doctors will complement the framework of clinical governance. Involvement in activities that fall within this framework at this stage will facilitate the transition to this new culture of regular reassessment of fitness to practise. This should ensure that the problems of underperformance are largely prevented but where they occur, clear strategies to manage these will include opportunities for retraining and education.

A similar philosophy could be applied to those tasks that are not seen in an explicitly educational context. The tasks that the PCG/PCT will have to undertake will provide a focus of learning opportunity in relation to clinical and organisational activity. The knowledge base will need to be consolidated, managerial and organisational skills developed. Again, this reflects the 'curriculum' that the Bolingbroke Group created for itself. In many ways the Bolingbroke Group mirrored the real world of the PCG/PCT that is now upon us.

Evaluation of the Bolingbroke model

The Bolingbroke Group was a unidisciplinary group learning activity for GPs and was established to tackle real concerns about the quality of general practice in Inner London. The group attempted to address some of the emotional and psychological pressures that can contribute to burn-out as well as specific training and educational needs in a more task-oriented way. Evaluating the success of the group proved difficult. Perhaps the tools we used – audit of change in clinical behaviour and questionnaires that examined psychological well-being – were not sensitive to the real changes that occurred. Perhaps any measure of success can only be gauged in the longer term. Certainly reductionist models of a quantitative nature will never fully capture the effect of being engaged in activities such as this. However, formative evaluation along the way and the narratives of those interviewed afterwards indicate that for the individuals concerned, the group had a profound effect.

Individual experiences and outcomes were varied but all group members acknowledged the value of having time out of the practice routine to reflect on their own experience and that of others. Some who might have drifted away from general practice altogether were able to gain refreshment and insight that gave rise to new opportunities. Reflective learning, the support of others, facilitation by a teaching team and the role of the group analyst were key elements in this process.

Demonstrating the development of skills and attitudes that feed in to a higher quality of care for patients is not easy but it is hard to believe that patients did not benefit from the activities of this group. Similarly, practices as a whole will have been exposed to new ideas and new ways of working if only as a result of the sharing of ideas and good practice.

One of the successful outcomes of the group, which was not clear in the short term, has been the different aspects of the professional development of members of the group.

A very significant increase in group members' involvement in activities related to general practice organisational development and medical education was generated. The range of activities include:

- primary care group board membership
- local medical committee (LMC) membership
- undergraduate teaching
- ongoing small group learning.

In fact, one local PCG has no fewer than four former members of the Bolingbroke Group on its board. As an individual example, one group member who had been contemplating a complete change of career, to that of barrister, is now his board's lead on IT and an active LCM member as well. Something happened somewhere!

Developing the model in PCGs/PCTs

There seems to be no obvious reason why this educational model should not be developed further within PCGs/PCTs and in a wider field of medical education that would address the needs of clinical governance, CPD, revalidation and doctors whose performance gives cause for concern. Similarly, there is no reason why the model should not be developed for other groups working in the PCG, both unidisciplinary and multidisciplinary.

Current concerns about the isolation of single-handed GPs could be addressed by setting up PCG/PCT-based educational groups for these GPs. Visiting practices in my role as clinical governance lead has made me aware of the degree of isolation that some GPs experience and the lack of support they feel has been offered to them in the past. My perception is that these GPs are often working in areas of deprivation with associated social and medical problems that most of us find unattractive. It is easy to see why they become the scapegoats when issues of underperformance are raised but the reality is that the NHS, both new and old, has created and allowed them to occupy this role. Those I have met would welcome the opportunity to engage in locally based group learning activities. Will the resources be made available to enable them to do this?

However, I would not see the Bolingbroke model as being applicable to struggling single-handers alone. Any group of GPs would benefit. There may be a strong case for encouraging this in particular for non-principals – locums, assistants and retainers – who are often the forgotten partners in the provision of primary care. If this group of GPs is to be in touch with the culture and medical standards of their PCG/PCT they need a vehicle that will allow them to do this. Doctors who have left general practice and are contemplating re-entry would almost certainly welcome locally based educational opportunities. At a time when there are serious problems relating to the recruitment and retention of doctors in certain areas, PCGs/PCTs should be taking a proactive role in this field.

In saying that any group of GPs would benefit from educational activity based on the Bolingbroke model, it may be that the system for revalidation will actively encourage this. Certainly group learning and practice-based learning appear high on the agenda. For those who are found to be underperforming, it would seem sensible to develop local models of remedial therapy where performance can be observed and reassessed in a GP's practice rather than removing the GP to some distant assessment and support centre.

In many ways some of the elements of group educational activity are already taking place, as they always have, unconsciously. For example, PCG boards bring together individuals from different cultural backgrounds – GPs, nurses, lay members, non-executive members of the health authority, management chief executives – who are learning to work together in a task-oriented fashion. Those boards that are doing this successfully have recognised the value of spending time working at the organisational development of the board itself. Similarly, subcommittees and 'task forces' that are working on more narrowly defined areas of activity are having to come to terms with the individual and organisational opportunities and constraints that their members bring with them. Egos and organisational agendas can easily sabotage the shared agenda. Defining these and making the issues explicit and open to negotiation can be a difficult and time-consuming task. Boards that leave the roles of leadership and decision making to charismatic and enthusiastic chairs and chief executives run the risk of creating person-dependent organisations that do not necessarily reflect the needs of the organisation and individuals within it as a whole. When these powerful leaders move on there may be a hiatus as those left behind are ill prepared to fill the gap.

Historically GPs have undertaken management tasks with little or no training. The complexity and size of the rapidly changing agenda that confronts PCGs/PCTs illustrate the need for GPs and others to be aware of the issues involved both for individuals, the PCG/PCT and the subgroups, within the context of political initiatives. Again, this is an aspect of the Bolingbroke Group's success that is difficult to evaluate but all its members would acknowledge a growth in their understanding of these issues. This is an area of knowledge and skill that must be developed further if GPs and other medical professional groups are to have an effective voice in guiding the future development of their PCG/PCT. This will be of particular importance as the structure of the board changes when a PCG moves to PCT status, bringing with it a greater range of responsibilities that will have major implications for a trust's education and training strategy.

In summary, I see the Bolingbroke model of education as having a potentially valuable role for the following groups at PCG/PCT level:

- any group of GPs
- GPs working as single-handers or in small practices
- non-principals – locums, assistants, retainers, GPs returning to practice
- doctors whose performance gives rise to concern
- other unidisciplinary groups
- multidisciplinary groups.

Summary

The pace of change for PCGs/PCTs is rapid and not necessarily in the interests of patients or those who seek to care for them. However, the 'New NHS' can be seen as part of a continuum of change that demands an ongoing reappraisal of the identity and roles of the individuals and groups that work within the organisation. Running in parallel with organisational changes has been a move toward making doctors more accountable for their behaviour and actions. Serious issues of underperformance and professional misconduct have called into question the profession's ability to regulate itself. Clinical governance and revalidation seek to define acceptable levels of performance for the NHS as a whole and for doctors working within it.

PCGs, for better or worse, are rapidly moving to trust status. In so doing they will have to recognise the implications that this has for supporting and developing their workforce. Clear strategies for education and training will need to be put in place which will have to meet the demands of clinical governance. Individual GPs will have to demonstrate their own fitness to practise. The resources for this aspect of development are unclear, as is the framework for ensuring the processes of revalidation. These issues are being grappled with both locally and nationally. There is a real danger that the outcome will be a process in which boxes are ticked, reports filed and little in the way of true professional development takes place. If a real shift in the way we educate and support ourselves is to occur then models akin to that of the Bolingbroke Group need to be developed. This model offers opportunities for GPs to undertake meaningful CPD and addresses many if not all the areas that are regarded as current best practice in this field. The model is applicable to a range of different groups. Underpinning its success is the 'support' role of the group.

While GPs express a willingness to embrace the principles of CPD and revalidation, in the interests of both patients and themselves, the government, not unlike its predecessors, pays lip service to the notion of support for doctors. Resources to fund a comprehensive programme of CPD remain unclear. Without proper resources both nationally and at PCG/PCT level, doctors will remain unsupported and patients may feel unprotected. Meanwhile, in a climate of increasing public accountability and medicolegal litigation, the question is not so much 'Can we afford to properly resource CME for GPs?' but 'Can we afford not to?'

If we fail to provide effective support to GPs and other members of the healthcare team we face the very real danger that individuals will succumb to the problems of stress, low morale and burnout that confronted the GPs entering the Bolingbroke Group.

Building upon some of the lessons exemplified by this group will be one way of avoiding these problems. More than that, this model will enable individuals to realise their true potential as a result of the support and inspiration that working together allows. Here is a model that allows individuals to identify their real educational needs in the context of the group. This mirrors the need for meaningful CPD for the individual working within a PCG/PCT. If we are serious about *Supporting Doctors, Protecting Patients* this is the type of model that needs to be developed.

Appendix: an example of a term's programme for the Bolingbroke Group 14.1.98–25.3.98

14.1.98 MEDICOLEGAL PROBLEMS
Dr Stephanie Bown from the Medical Protection Society

A series of questions generated by the group were addressed by Dr Bown leading in to a discussion that highlighted the medicolegal threat that is felt by all group members.

21.1.98 MENTAL HEALTH ISSUES
Dr Alan Cohen, Research Fellow at the Sainsbury's Foundation

Management of schizophrenia and other chronic mental illness in the community was discussed. Handouts and booklets outlined guidelines and provided feedback on research into this area in which several group members had been involved. Attention to the physical needs of patients with mental health problems was highlighted. Various aspects of counselling were debated.

28.1.98 CARDIOLOGY UPDATE
Dr Vasadevi from the Dept of Cardiology at St George's

Current management of common cardiovascular problems was discussed, again using a series of questions previously generated by the group. The fact that our speaker had previously worked in general practice meant that his approach was attuned to the real needs of group members and this was commented upon.

4.2.98 COPING WITH CHANGE
Dr Howard Freeman, local GP and non-executive member of the health authority

Presentation of the White Paper *The New NHS* and discussion of the implications of this with particular attention paid to the formation of primary care groups. Focus on what is happening in MSW Health Authority.

11.2.98 MEDICAL GENETICS
Dr Murday from the Dept of Genetics at St George's

This session addressed some clinical issues and some local service issues. Both were helpful to the group who felt that this is an area of medicine that has moved on rapidly in recent years. All acknowledged difficulty in keeping up to date in this field and were grateful for an update on recent developments.

4.3.98 CAREER DEVELOPMENT
What are the options?
Andy Morgan

Development of special interests within and without general practice
Contributions from the whole group who have a wide range of experience

Financial planning
Representative from the BMA

An interactive day with group members sharing their own experiences that included involvement in teaching (both undergraduate and postgraduate), occupational health, public health, sports medicine, nursing home medical officer, LMC involvement, advisers to health authority, etc.

The financial planning session focused on pensions and highlighted the lack of financial planning among the group members, leaving us all with much to take away and ponder.

11.3.98 THE PRACTICE NURSE
Kate Hawley, GP with special interest in the role of nursing in primary care

Areas covered included the future role of the practice nurse, the role of the nurse practitioner, and the integrated nursing team. Group members contributed information about the range of activities that their own practice nurses were involved in. The differences between practices provoked much useful discussion and gave members new ideas for innovation in their own practices.

18.3.98 PAEDIATRIC UPDATE
Immunisation update
Dr David Elliman, Community Paediatrician

New developments in paediatric care
Dr Thurlbeck from the Dept of Paediatrics at St George's

The immunisation update was particularly welcomed as it coincided with the latest 'scare' concerning the MMR vaccine. A good example of the value of evidence-based medicine being brought into action.

Dr Thurlbeck addressed a series of questions that the group had generated and the clinical update was appreciated by all. Accompanied by useful handouts on management of some common paediatric problems in practice.

25.3.98 FINAL SESSION – REVIEW OF THE COURSE AND FUTURE PLANS
Evaluation and feedback session
Options for further learning
Developing a portfolio – for the individual and the group.

The term's activities were reviewed by the group and there was common agreement that much had been learnt. The benefits of doing this in a group were acknowledged. The combination of support as exemplified by the Gerhard sessions and the task-oriented approach of the topic sessions was seen as a useful model for further work. However, the reality of life beyond LIZEI is that there would not be the same amount of 'protected time' available and group members wondered how realistic it would be to try and continue.

Despite these anxieties, all but two members made a commitment to meet on a Wednesday afternoon to continue the group learning activity. We opted to try the 'puns and dens' model with a view to identifying our educational needs.

The idea of developing a learning portfolio will be further explored as part of our personal development plans.

References

Balint E and Norell J (eds) (1973) *Six Minutes for the Patient: interactions in general practice consultations*. Tavistock, London.

Balint E *et al.* (1993) *The Doctor, The Patient and The Group: Balint revisited*. Routledge, London.

Binney G, Wilke G and Craft M (1995) *The Acceptance and Shaping of Change: health promotion in primary care*. St George's Medical School, London.

Bion W (1961) *Experiences in Groups*. Tavistock/Routledge, London.

Bolas C (1994) *Being a Character: psychoanalysis and self experience*. Routledge, London.

Bourdieu P (1977) *Outline of a Theory of Practice*. Cambridge University Press, Cambridge.

Bowie M (1991) *Lacan*. Fontana, London.

Bowlby J (1981) *Attachment (vol 1), Separation (vol 2), Loss (vol 3)*. Penguin, Harmondsworth.

Casey D (1993) *Managing Learning in Organisations*. Open University Press, Buckingham, pp 19–31, 69–85.

DoH (1998) *A First Class Service*. Department of Health, London.

Department of Health (1999) *Supporting Doctors, Protecting Patients*. Department of Health, London.

Elias N (1978) *The Civilising Process*. Blackwell, Oxford.

Foulkes S (1986) *Group-Analytic Psychotherapy*. Karnac, London.

Geertz C (1993) *The Interpretation of Cultures*. Fontana, London.

Giddens A (1999) *A Runaway World: how globalisation is reshaping our lives*. Profile, London.

Handy C (1994) *The Empty Raincoat: making sense of the future*. Hutchinson, London.

Hirschhorn L (1993) *The Workplace Within: psychodynamics of organisational life*. MIT Press, Cambridge MA.

Höffe O (1981) *Klassiker der Philosophie II: von Immanuel Kant bis Jean-Paul Sartre*. Verlag CH Beck, Munich, pp 62–93.

Hopper E (1999) The social unconscious in clinical work. In: C Oakley (ed) *What is a Group? A new look at theory in practice*. Rebus, London, pp 112–47.

Hughes E (1984) *The Sociological Eye*. Transaction, New Brunswick, p 399.

Kets de Vries F (1993) *Leaders, Fools and Imposters: essays on the psychology of leadership*. Jossey-Bass, San Francisco.

Klein M (1963) *Our Adult World and its Roots in Infancy*. Hogarth, London.

Kohut H (1971) *The Analysis of the Self*. International Universities Press, New York.

Lasch C (1979) *The Culture of Narcissism*. Norton, New York.

Leach E (1986) *Social Anthropology*. Fontana, Glasgow.

Obholzer A and Roberts V (1994) *The Unconscious at Work: individual and organisational stress in the human services*. Routledge, London.

Pollock G (1980) Ageing or aged: development or pathology. In: G Pollock and S Greenspan (eds) *The Course of Lives*. NIHM, Bethesda.

Redle F (1945) *Group Emotions and Leadership, vol* 5. Psychiatry Press, New York, pp 15–22.

Schmidbauer W (1993) *Hilflose Helfer: über die seelische Problematik der helfenden Berufe*. Rowohlt, Hamburg.

Skynner R and Cleese J (1993) *Life and How to Survive It*. Methuen, London.

Tustin F (1986) *Autistic Barriers in Neurotic Patients*. Karnac, London.

van der Kleij G (1982) About the matrix. *Group Analysis*. **15**(3): 219.

Weber M (1963) *Selections From His Work* (with introduction by SM Miller). Crowell, New York.

Winnicott D (1965) *The Maturational Processes and the Facilitating Environment: studies in the theory of emotional development*. Hogarth Press, London.

Wittgenstein L (1997) *Philosophical Investigation*. Blackwell, Oxford.

Yalom I (1980) *Existential Psychotherapy*. Basic Books, New York.

Zinkin L (1983) Malignant mirroring. *Group Analysis*. **16**(2): 113–26.

Further reading

Barnes B, Ernst S and Hyde K (1999) *An Introduction to Groupwork: a group-analytic perspective*. Macmillan, London.

Binney G and Williams C (1995) *Leaning into the Future: changing the way people change organisations*. Brearley, London.

Bocock R (1978) *Freud and Modern Society*. Holmes and Meier, New York.

Brookfield S (1986) *Understanding and Facilitating Adult Learning*. Open University Press, Milton Keynes.

Burkitt I (1991) *Social Selves: theories of the social formation of personality*. Sage, London.

Calman K (1998) *A Review of Continuing Professional Development in General Practice: a report by the Chief Medical Officer*. Department of Health, London.

Carrithers M (1992) *Why Humans Have Cultures: explaining anthropology and social diversity*. Oxford University Press, Oxford.

Cohen A (1995) *The Symbolic Construction of Community*. Routledge, London.

De Geus A (1999) *The Living Company: growth, learning and longevity in business*. Brearley, London.

Elder A and Samule O (eds) (1987) *'While I'm Here, Doctor': a study of the doctor–patient relationship*. Tavistock/Routledge, London.

Erikson E (1959) *Identity and the Life Cycle*. International Universities Press, New York.

Freud A (1937) *The Ego and the Mechanisms of Defence*. Hogarth, London.

Freud S (1972) *Two Short Accounts of Psycho-Analysis*. Penguin, Harmondsworth.

Frosch S (1991) *Identity Crisis, Modernity, Psychoanalysis and the Self*. Macmillan, Basingstoke.

Giddens A (1997) *Modernity and Self-Identity*. Polity Press, Bristol.

Glass N (1996) *Management Masterclass*. Brearley, London.

Good B (1997) *Medicine, Rationality and Experience*. Cambridge University Press, Cambridge.

Hildebrand P (1995) *Beyond Mid-Life Crisis: a psychodynamic approach to ageing*. Sheldon, London.

Jarvis P (1995) *Adult and Continuing Education*. Routledge, London.

Kets de Vries F and Miller V (1989) *The Neurotic Organisation: diagnosing and changing counterproductive styles of management*. Jossey-Bass, London.

Morgan G (1986) *Images of Organization*. Sage, London.

NHSE (1999) *Clinical Governance: quality in the new NHS*. Department of Health, London.

Ohmae K (1992) *The Borderless World: power and strategy in the global marketplace*. Harper Collins, London.

Pedler M (1983) *Action Learning in Practice*. Gower, Guildford.

Pedler M, Burgoyne J and Boydell T (1996) *The Learning Company*. McGraw-Hill, London.

Phillips A (1988) *Winnicott*. Fontana, London.

Roland M and Baker R (1999) *Clinical Governance: a practical guide for primary care teams*. National Primary Care Research and Development Centre, University of Manchester.

Royal College of General Practitioners, General Practitioners Committee (1999) *Good Medical Practice for General Practitioners*. Draft document for consultation. RCGP/GPC, London.

Royal College of General Practitioners, General Practitioners Committee (1999) *Revalidation for Clinical General Practice*. Draft document for consultation. RCGP/GPC, London.

Rudnytsky P (ed) (1993) *Transitional Objects and Potential Spaces: literary uses of DW Winnicott*. Columbia, New York.

Secretary of State for Health (1997) *The New NHS: modern, dependable*. Department of Health, London.

Sharpe M (ed) (1995) *The Third Eye: supervision of analytic groups*. Macmillan, London.

Sinclair S (1997) *Making Doctors: an institutional apprenticeship*. Berg, Oxford.

Stacey R (1992) *Managing Chaos*. Kogan Page, London.

Stapley F (1996) *The Personality of the Organisation: a psycho-dynamic explanation of culture and change*. Free Association, London.

Wolf E (1988) *Treating the Self: elements of clinical self-psychology*. Guilford, New York.

INDEX